OUTPERFORM THE NORM

for
METABOLISM MASTERY

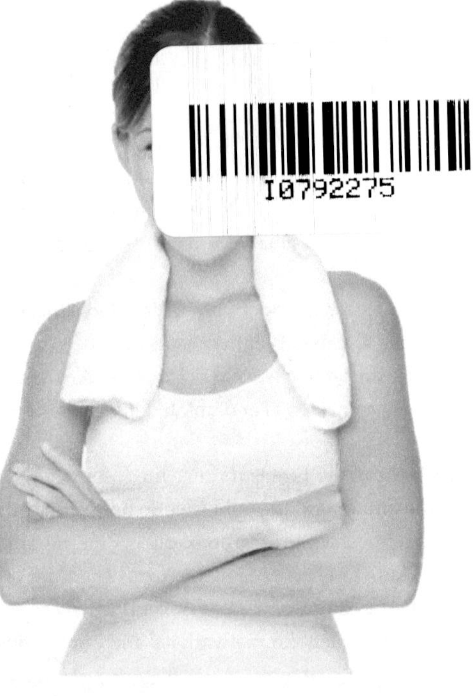

A Simple

8 STEP PLAN:
Diet Less. Eat More.
Lose Weight for LIFE

SCOTT WELLE | *#1 Best Selling Author*

To everyone who wants to live healthier and have a better
relationship with food, but has been confused by misinformation,
this one's for you.

Introduction

This is a serious book about weight loss. It's not based on fads, gimmicks, quick fixes or the latest crazy trend. This book is about healthy, sustainable, long-term weight loss done the *right way*.

What I'm going to reveal in the following chapters is my unfiltered, zero-BS 8-step plan that I use to help clients lose weight...and keep it off. Some of it will make you nod, some of it will make you shake your head and some of it will have you saying, "Did he *really* just say that?"

Enter *The Gap* (no, I'm not talking about the store). The Gap is the difference between what we KNOW and what we actually DO. We live in a Google-ized society where information is so abundantly available that it often paralyzes us from action. Or more simply stated, it paralyzes us from taking the *correct action*. Unfortunately, information does not equal wisdom. Most people know that fresh fruit is healthier than fresh cheesecake but this doesn't stop them from ordering the latter dessert.

This book is going to deal more with doing than knowing. Massive action is the only thing that gets results. Nothing else. Massive intelligence with no action leaves you still battling the scale. And you deserve to see results.

I want you to know this going in so you're fully prepared. If you're looking for a book that will coax and coddle you and tell you it's going to be easy, this may not be the book for you. I only know how to write one way and I have to stay true to that. I hope you understand.

So, if you're ready and committed to making a change, *once and for all*, then please read on.

THE NORM	OUTPERFORM
HOPEFULLY	DEFINITELY
WHEN I HAVE TIME	I'LL MAKE IT A PRIORITY
EXCUSES	ACCOUNTABILITY
I HAVE TO	I GET TO
COMFORTABLE	CHALLENGED
SECURE DECISIONS	CALCULATED RISKS
SOMEDAY	TODAY
GIVEN	EARNED
EASY WAY	BEST WAY
RESOURCES	RESOURCEFULNESS
PLAY NOT TO LOSE	PLAY TO WIN
FOCUSED ON ME	FOCUSED ON WE
FOLLOWER	LEADER

TABLE OF CONTENTS

How to Use This Book

This is a start-to-finish type of book. Each chapter builds on the one that preceded it. If you're looking to get the most out of this book, then start at the beginning and work your way through.

Two important notes on how to get maximum benefit from this book:

1. Do the action plans at the end of each chapter! Perhaps this seems blatantly obvious to you but you'd be surprised how many people will read a book and never the necessary actions to see results. I know how this is—I've been there myself. I've just wanted to read the book and when the author asked me to do something, I just said "that's okay, I don't *really* need to do that. I can do it later." And I ended up getting nowhere.

Please take the time to complete the action plans. A very small amount of time invested on the front end will pay off in huge results on the back end.

2. Either create your own "Commitment Contract" (you'll find out what this is later) or go to **OutperformTheNorm.com/books** to access the one I've created for you. Once you've downloaded it, print it off and get started. But please do this *before* you do anything else. Almost all of your action plans are specifically geared towards refining your commitment contract and making it

the best it can be. It's truly a "working document" throughout this book. There are many other helpful tools and downloads included as well.

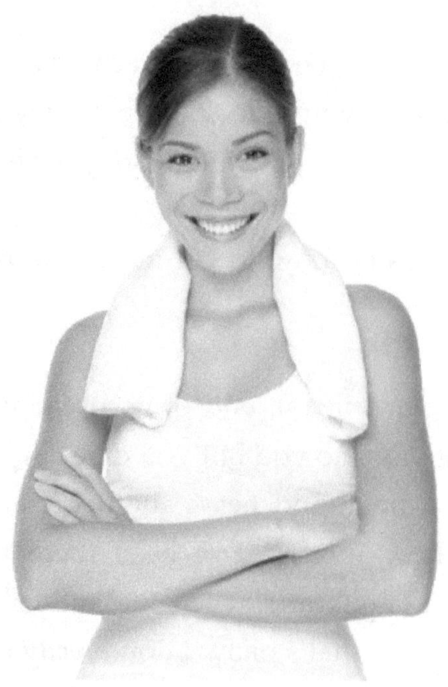

OutperformTheNorm.com/books

Let's get started!

Scott

The OUTPERFORMER'S Creed

Outperforming isn't a destination.
IT'S A WAY OF LIFE.

You'll never **FEEL READY** for something you **HAVEN'T DONE**

BE A PILLAR OF POSITIVITY

You have *enough time* for your priorities,
WHAT ARE THEY?

LIGHTEN UP, LAUGH AT YOUR IMPERFECTIONS

Why Not **YOU?**
CHANGE ≠ **WORSE**

WE > ME EMBRACE **THE SUCK**

Look up from your phone **and greet a stranger.** THEY'RE SOMEBODY.

YOU'RE WORTH IT

GIVE AND YOU SHALL RECEIVE

PAY THE PRICE OF **ADMISSION**

OVERNIGHT SUCCESS TAKES *years* OF HARD WORK.

SMILE. ■
■ **SWEAT.**
SERVE. ■

FUEL YOUR BODY, NOURISH YOUR BRAIN

HIGH achievement & fulfillment **ARE MEANT TO GO hand-in-hand**

Make the most of your precious days on this planet

Never put **OTHERS DOWN** to pull you up

Let your **WEIRDO LIGHT** shine bright

LEAVE A LEGACY

Strive for **PROGRESS,** *not perfection*

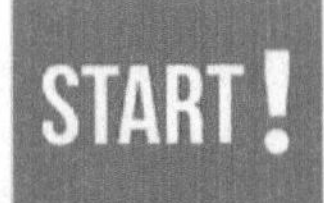

PLAY **TO WIN**

TAKE NOTHING FOR GRANTED

BE WHO YOU SAY **YOU ARE**

BRING THE JOY LAY **ONE** BRICK **EVERYDAY**

LEADERS ARE **READERS.**
LEARNERS ARE **EARNERS.**

THERE IS NO FAILURE *only feedback*

IT WON'T BE EASY BUT IT WILL BE WORTH IT

Have **FUN.**
Take **RISKS.**
Love **PEOPLE.**

BE DRIVEN BY **DESIRE,** NOT PARALYZED **BY FEAR**

START!

NO GOAL IS TOO LOFTY IF YOU HAVE AN INTELLIGENT PLAN *to accomplish it*

LISTEN AND ACCEPT OTHERS, even when their opinions differ from yours

THE GREATEST PRESENT IS YOUR PRESENCE

Self-limiting beliefs ARE THE GOVERNOR ON YOUR POTENTIAL

Don't wait until someday. **DO IT NOW!**

SUCCESS IS A TEAM SPORT

CHOOSE AN ATTITUDE OF **GRATITUDE**

STEP IT UP. Today is game day.

CHAPTER 1
ATTITUDE

"Control the Controllables."

Before we even talk about a single exercise, calorie or portion size, we're going to talk about the most important asset in anything you're trying to accomplish – your attitude. Yes, ATTITUDE. If you don't have 100% belief that this time you're going to be able to get it done, then please don't read any further. All the strategies in the world can't overcome self-doubt and apprehension.

Studies have shown that highly confident people react differently in the aspect of *permanence*. In a nutshell, permanence means that if something negative has happened to you, do you believe that it will be a PERMANENT result...meaning that it will continue to happen again?

In this case, I'm speaking to anyone who has ever tried a weight loss plan and failed. If this is you, LET IT GO. It's in the past. Done. Over. Good riddance. It is NOT a *permanent* result.

Thinking that negative history is condemned to repeat itself ruins confidence and self-belief. We need to start fresh.

Now that your mind is clear, here are the other critical components of a successful weight loss attitude...

Be Disgusted

Right now you could be one of two people:

Option A: You aren't that happy with the way you look and how your body feels and you'd "kind of like to" lose weight.

Option B: You're disgusted with the way you look, hate the way you feel and have a burning desire to lose weight.

Which one do you think has the best chance for success? You guessed it – Option B.

Believe it or not, your own personal level of disgust with your current situation is a powerful determinant to whether you accomplish something. People who are disgusted with their weight will take greater actions to lose weight. People who are disgusted with their financial situation will take greater actions to gain wealth. It's that simple. This applies almost universally to any area of life.

Please know I'm not advocating that you beat yourself up psychologically for your present condition. There's a difference between being disgusted with your current *situation* and being disgusted with yourself as a *person.* I never want you to diminish your intrinsic value as a person. That NEVER works out positively.

What I AM saying is, the deeper the level of your discontent for your current circumstances, the better off you will be. If you're reading this thinking that you're not *that* disgusted, it is actually something you can *create.* Go put on something that you used to be able to wear but is now skin-tight. Think of activities you used to be able to participate in that you can no longer do. Hold up pictures of yourself when you were at your ideal weight side-by-side with a picture of you currently. Go ahead – do it!

How does that make you feel? Hopefully pretty disgusted.

Now, after you do these things, *use it as fuel for your motivational fire!* Don't do what everyone else does where they sulk and play the "woe is me" card. Let it create the burning desire that you need to make a powerful, lasting change. The purpose of this is

NOT to make you feel worse about yourself. The purpose of having you do this is to create an emotionally charged burning desire to change. Once you have this, you're unstoppable.

Unwavering Commitment To Your Goal

Before you embark on any great journey you need to commit to reaching the destination.

Funny, as I write this, I think about the movie *Point Break* (it was on TV last night) with Keanu Reeves. There's the part where all the surfers are sitting around the fire talking about how surfing requires total commitment because "you can't just turn back if you don't like the way things are going." This is the type of committed attitude you need to have towards weight loss. Will it be hard? Yes. Will you come across obstacles? Yes. Will it be worth it in the end? YES.

The best way to signify a commitment is to put it in writing. It's like any contract you sign. So take out a pen and paper (RIGHT NOW – don't wait) and write down the following on your commitment contract:

I, **[insert name],** am COMMITTED to losing (insert number of pounds) by (insert date). I will NOT turn back, even if I don't like the way things are going. I WILL succeed.

[Insert signature]

Make sure you sign it at the bottom! This makes the "commitment contract" more real than anything else you can do. And keep it handy – we'll be expanding on it later.

*If you did not download and print off your commitment contract you can make your own, but for simplicity's sake I'd highly recommend downloading the one I've created for you at **OutperformTheNorm.com/books.**

Shaping Your Environment

First, did you really write out your commitment contract? If you haven't, PLEASE don't go any farther until this is done.

Most people don't realize that it takes the same amount of energy to do successful, constructive things as it does unsuccessful, unconstructive things. You may not believe this but it's the truth. Or at least it *should* be.

Here's why it's take more energy for most people to be successful – they have not properly "shaped their environment." This concept comes from a book called *Switch* and it absolutely applies to weight loss. Shaping your environment involves putting the pieces in place to make success as EASY as possible for you. What a novel concept!

What am I talking about here? Please consider some of these examples:

You find it hard to resist cookies and sweets when you're at home: Don't have cookies and sweets at home. Clear out your cupboards.

You try to exercise but workouts frequently get missed: Either a) schedule it like you would any other meeting and *stick to it*, or b) workout first thing in the morning before life can get in the way.

You find it hard to drink enough water: Have a water bottle on you at all times. Or throw a case of water in your car. Or purposely walk past the drinking fountain on your breaks.

You never have time to eat breakfast: Cook it the night before or have a healthy bar or shake ready that you can grab-and-go with in the morning.

Some of these things may seem painfully obvious to you but they're not for a lot of people. Don't make it more difficult than it needs to be. Part of your attitude needs to be spending a certain amount of time genuinely *thinking* about how you can best shape your environment for success. Make it as easy as possible on yourself.

Crystal Clear Clarity

Where are you going? Don't tell me a state, or a county, or a city, or a neighborhood – I want the *specific address*. I want to know exactly where you're going.

Look at weight loss the same way. When you have crystal clear clarity on your destination, you have set your GPS. Once we have identified the plan (discussed later) you are effectively following the turn-by-turn directions. And when this is done you stand an unbelievably high chance for success.

It is very difficult to get where you want to go if you don't know where that is. How will you know if you're on track? How will you know if you're off course?

Sometimes I have clients tell me they want to get in shape. I say, "that's great – *round* is a shape. What exact shape are you looking for?" The more precisely you can describe exactly where you want to go, the better chance you have of arriving there. Don't be afraid to use your imagination...and when you do so, imagine every aspect of your life in *vivid detail* being enhanced through your weight loss. Your imagination has great power to become reality.

Resiliency

Remember that GPS we were discussing in the last point? I'll let you in on a little secret – you're STILL going to take a wrong turn and start heading in the wrong direction at some point. We all do it. Accept it.

I've been in the health and fitness industry for 12+ years and I've NEVER seen someone do everything perfectly, all the time, regardless of what they're trying to accomplish. Everyone gets knocked down. What matters is that you get back up. But thinking that you're going to go through your entire weight loss journey without any obstacles or adversity is not only naïve – it's *insane*.

Sorry, but it's true.

The reason I'm bringing this up is that I want to caution you against adopting a perfectionistic, all-or-nothing attitude. The people who do this are the ones who see unbelievable results in a short period of time. Many people are capable of buckling down in the short term...but this never lasts. At SOME point there will be a slip up. And the person with this dichotomous mindset typically doesn't know how to respond when their plan is not perfect. They're either on it or off it. And when they're off it, they're usually waaaay off it.

A much better approach is to actually anticipate adversity and setbacks...and know how to respond to them when they come. From a weight loss perspective, you're going to miss a workout. You're going to eat a piece of cheesecake. Big deal - these things happen. And you can either let them totally derail you or you can just accept them for what they are, move on and start fresh. Don't punish yourself or berate your own ego. Just move on. Even if it happened once doesn't mean it will be a *permanent* result.

Attitude Action Plan

Please do not overlook the importance of having the proper attitude. It astounds me the number of weight loss and diet books I see that fail to address this key component. Everybody wants to deal with the ABC's of calories and exercise (which are important, and will be discussed later), but unless your attitude is in the right spot going in, you're doomed for failure. With the proper attitude, however, you're armed for success.

Before moving onto *Amounts*, here is your *Attitude Action Plan*:

1. Write your commitment contract (please tell me you've done this already!) and keep it in a visible area so you will see it daily. On the bathroom mirror, on the fridge, on the nightstand or in the car are all good examples. Take a picture of it with your phone and use it as your Home Screen or Lock Screen. This will keep reminded of the commitment you've made.

2. On your commitment contract, write down something about your current situation that disgusts you. Directly below this next to "Improving this will," write how your life will improve if you improve your current situation.

Example:

I'm disgusted by: My current weight and low energy levels

Improving this will: Make me happier and be a better person for my friends and family

The more examples you can personally come up with, the better. At the bare minimum try to come up with 3. Take which one is the most significant to you and write it on your commitment contract.

3. Think about ways you can shape the environment to make success easy. What does this look like for you? Setting out your workout clothes the night before? Clearing out your cupboards and fridge? Preparing meals in advance? Try to come up with at least 3 ways that you can make your journey to success easier and write them on your commitment contract.

4. Decide what you're going to tell yourself when you make a mistake. I'm not talking about punishment – I'm talking about something constructive that you can say to yourself that will allow you to immediately put it behind you, refocus and start fresh. It can be something as simple as saying the word "fresh," or go back and rewrite your commitment contract, which will truly make it feel like you're starting anew.

CHAPTER 2
AMOUNTS

"There are no 'Good' Foods or 'Bad' Foods...
in Right Amounts."

This chapter will discuss the *amount* of food you're actually eating (in terms of number of calories). If you don't know exactly how much food (fuel) you should be taking in, it's virtually impossible to determine how long it will take to get to your goal. It may be days...it may be weeks. You may not get there altogether!

I don't think it's any great secret that America is a supersized country. Studies have shown that, not only have the plates that we eat on substantially increased in size over the past 20 years, so have the portion sizes (increasing by roughly 25%, on average). Combine this will less overall activity in our lifestyle and that's why we are where we are.

Bottom line – we're eating more and we're moving less. If our society could find a way to reverse these two things, books like this one wouldn't be necessary. I'd have to start writing cheesy romance novels!

(No one wants that)

Most of our overconsumption of calories comes from the fact that we've lost the ability to judge portion sizes. We're a value-driven culture. We want more food for our dollar. And this has hurt our waistlines.

A good rule of them when looking at portion sizes is that a portion of lean protein is about the size of the palm of your hand and a portion of carbohydrates is the size of your clenched fist. If you're used to eating much more than this, it is probably because you've gotten used to overly large portion sizes.

Controlling portion sizes and having a good approximation of the number of calories you should be taking in on a daily basis is essential to any weight loss program. Because we all have unique bodies and genetics, there is always going to be an *art* to any weight loss program. But, by breaking down your individual daily caloric intake we are making it much more of a *science* (a good thing).

Determining Your Calories Intake

The most longstanding formula to determine individual caloric requirement comes from the *Harris-Benedict Formula*. It gives the best approximation of your calorie expenditure on a daily basis.

Here are the formulas:

Women: BMR = 655 + (4.35 x weight in pounds) + (4.7 x height in inches) - (4.7 x age in years)

Men: BMR = 66 + (6.23 x weight in pounds) + (12.7 x height in inches) - (6.8 x age in years)

Yes, I know the equations are somewhat complex but they are the best out there. Please use a calculator and write down your number.

These formulas are determining your BMR, or *Basal Metabolic Rate*. Your BMR is the baseline number of calories your body needs daily to maintain basic physiological functioning. In other words, if you were to wake up and do nothing other than lie on the couch all day, your BMR is the number of calories your body needs to do this and *maintain* your weight.

However, I'm assuming everyone reading this book is doing something other than lying on the couch all day, so we need to add in an additional lifestyle component.

So, take your BMR number and multiply it by the following:

- ✓ Sedentary (little or no exercise): BMR x 1.2
- ✓ Lightly active (light exercise/sports 1-3 days/week): BMR x 1.375
- ✓ Moderately active (moderate exercise/sports 3-5 days/week): BMR x 1.55
- ✓ Very active (hard exercise/sports 6-7 days a week): BMR x 1.725
- ✓ Extra active (very hard exercise/sports & physical job or 2x training): BMR x 1.9

Write your total number down.

These numbers are adding in the *activity component* to your lifestyle. It makes sense – the more active you are on a daily basis, the more calories you will require. The resultant number from multiplying your BMR x your activity factor is the number of calories you would need to take in to *maintain your bodyweight*.

I'll say this on the equation - I've seen hundreds of people complete this over the years and most people want to overestimate their activity component. Please don't do this. If you try to exercise 3 times per week but you usually miss at least one workout, you are not in the "moderately active" category. We're not going off *targets*; we're going off *actuals*. Be honest with where you are so we can come up with a realistic number. It will benefit you more in the long term.

Lastly, if you're someone who exercises regularly and you do so with a heart rate monitor (a device that tells you how hard your heart is beating during cardiovascular exercise, discussed in the Bonus section), you can add in those numbers to your BMR instead of using the activity factor. For example, if you walk on the treadmill for 30 minutes everyday and you know you burn 250 calories on average, just add this onto your BMR to determine your total maintenance caloric intake.

Creating a Caloric Deficit

Now that you know how many calories you need to take in on a daily basis to maintain weight, let's determine how many calories you should be taking in to lose weight.

Just so we're clear, a caloric deficit means you're burning more calories each day than you're taking in, which will lead to weight loss. A caloric surplus means you're taking in more calories than you're burning, which will lead to weight gain.

Perhaps you've heard that one pound = 3500 calories. This means that, to lose one pound, we need to create a caloric deficit of 3500 calories (obviously, we're not talking about doing this in one day!). There are two ways to do this – either decrease your calories or increase your activity (or a combination of both). Right now we'll focus on calories but the key is to create a systematic approach that will not have you over restricting your calories so that your metabolism slows down, your body starts eating its lean muscle for fuel and, in turn, retains your stored body fat.

Here are three good examples of safe weight loss strategies:

- ✓ Daily caloric deficit of 250 calories per day = about 2-3 pounds per month

- ✓ Daily caloric deficit of 500 calories per day = about 4-5 pounds per month

- ✓ Daily caloric deficit of 1000 calories per day = about 8-9 pounds per month

(Don't worry; we will be going into the types of foods and combinations later)

Now, I'm onto you. I'll bet that you're looking at these numbers and thinking the first two options are just TOO SLOW and that you want to lose weight as fast as possible. And that's fine. I get it. We're a society of instant gratification. But I want you to look at your weight loss LONG TERM. The death of many diets is the over restriction of calories. Here's why:

Most people don't realize, when you over restrict your calories, you're actually ruining your metabolism because you're slowing down your metabolic rate. Your body thinks it's starving. It is critical that you find the balance between creating a caloric deficit that will facilitate weight loss and not crossover into the area where your metabolism slows. This is why, for those who habitually diet this way, the weight is usually gained back at some point...and then some.

Hydration

Our society is chronically dehydrated. We drink too little water and too much soda, energy drink, coffee, and other caffeinated beverages. This daily routine creates an imbalance between products that suck water out and those that put water back in.

Water is critically important for some of the following reasons:

- ✓ Improved mental clarity
- ✓ Improved digestion and absorption of nutrients
- ✓ Less back and joint pain
- ✓ Reduced risk of cancer
- ✓ Improved flexibility
- ✓ More energy
- ✓ Detoxifies the body

I'm astounded how few people actually drink enough water in their daily lives. A study in the *European Journal of Clinical Nutrition* showed that losing 1-2% of your bodyweight in dehydration has a corresponding 2-3% decrease in performance. And this performance can be in MANY areas, from cognitive functioning, to mental alertness, to reaction time, to the ability of the muscles to contract and relax and to general overall fatigue. Dehydration affects people not only athletically but also in their everyday lives.

Think about this point for a second. I currently weigh about 185, which means that if I lose 2-3 pounds of my bodyweight through perspiration (sweating) or respiration (breathing), I'm already dehydrated and not performing at my best. The hydration window is THAT small. And 2-3 pounds can happen in a blink of an eye, with you barely even realizing it's happening.

So, how much water is the right amount?

I advocate we drink a *minimum* of half our body weight in ounces of water, daily. So, if you weigh 128 pounds, eight 8-ounce glasses is a good starting point. If you weigh 150 pounds you should target 75 ounces, and if you weigh 200 pounds you should target 100 ounces.

Ounces of water daily = half of your body weight (in pounds)

If this seems like an obnoxiously large amount of water relative to what you're currently consuming, that's ok. *Work up to it!* Just focus on steadily increasing your water each week and you'll be there before you know it. Yes, you'll be in the bathroom more often than you are now...but it will be more than worth it. From a weight loss standpoint, this is why:

The brain control centers for thirst and hunger are next to each other and often these things can be confused. We THINK we're hungry but we're actually just thirsty. Drinking more water can help you distinguish whether your body is *genuinely* hungry. The best way to keep a handle on thirst and hunger is to drink small amounts of water, frequently, throughout the day.

Drinking water and remaining hydrated also helps control portion sizes and overeating. If your stomach has the right amount of water in it you'll be less likely to overeat. Again, having small amounts of water regularly throughout the day will maximize the chances that your portion sizes are appropriate for you.

Amounts Action Plan

This chapter is where the rubber meets the road and we start to look at your weight loss from a scientific standpoint. Now that we have the best approximation of how many calories you should be taking in daily to maintain weight, we can create a structured plan for success.

Here is your action plan:

1. Go back to your commitment contract. To reach your goal weight by your goal date, what is the caloric deficit that you would need to create DAILY to achieve this? If you're not the best with math, you can use the following:

- ✓ How many weeks in the future is your goal date? Write it down.
- ✓ How many pounds are you going to lose by this date? Write it down.
- ✓ Now, the number of weeks divided by the number of pounds = the number of pounds you will lose per week. Write it down.
- ✓ Take the number of pounds per week x 3500. Write it down.
- ✓ Take this number and divide it by 7. Write it down. This number is the caloric deficit you'd need to create daily

through nutrition and exercise to be able to achieve your goal.

As an example, I want to lose 5 pounds in 8 weeks. Dividing the pounds by the weeks means I'm losing an average of .625 pounds per week. When I multiply this by 3500, I need to have a caloric deficit of 2,187.5 calories per week, and dividing this by 7 means I need a caloric deficit of 312.5 calories daily.

Remember, the maximum caloric deficit you should have each day is 1,000 calories! If your numbers come out to any more than this daily, it would be in your best interest to revise it to something more realistic. Could you go more than 1,000 calories if you *really* needed to? Yes, I'm sure you could. But you stand the best chance of LONG TERM success by capping it at a maximum of 1,000.

2. Determine your daily ounces of water you need each day (hopefully you've done this already) and write it on your commitment contract.

The next step is to assess the number of ounces of water you're *currently* taking in. How far are you from your goal number of ounces? Better yet, what actions will you need to take and how can you shape the environment to close this gap? Try to make it as simple as possible. It could be an extra glass of water with each meal you have or taking breaks at work to stop by the drinking fountain. But come up with a realistic routine you can execute to hit your goal hydration each day.

CHAPTER 3
FOODS AND FUELS

"Fuel Your Body to Outperform."

If you've read any of my other books you know that I don't think of food as food. Food is FUEL. And I'm not going to change my analogy for this book. Why should I? Every single calorie you shove into your mouth brings about a given result. Just like Newton's law – every action causes a reaction. And the foods you eat are directly responsible for not only your weight, but also how you feel and for a given energy output.

Simply look at food like the gas you put in your car. You put high quality fuel into your car, it's going to burn cleaner, last longer and function better. You put in garbage for fuel you can expect your car to run like garbage. Your body is no different.

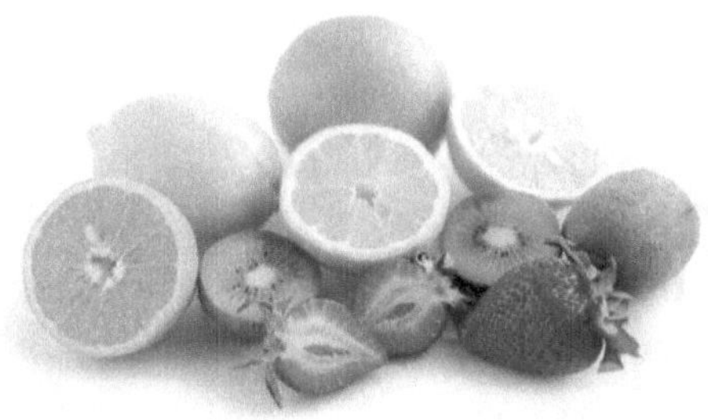

Have you ever heard the phrase *"you are what you eat?"*

It's absolutely true and this is why:

Your body is CONSTANTLY replacing itself...all the way down to the cellular level. This turnover cycle happens much faster than you probably realize. This is the average amount of time it takes for some of your tissues and organs to completely replace itself:

Skin: 2-4 weeks
Liver: 5 months

Taste buds: 10 days
Lungs: 2-3 weeks
Stomach lining: 2-3 days

Other than certain areas of your brain, every single area of your body will be rebuilt and be completely different in 8-10 years (including your bones!). Amazing.

Why am I telling you this? Because if your body is constantly replacing itself and you're looking to build a better body (I sometimes refer to it as your "machine"), what would you like to build it out of - pastries and soda and cheeseburgers? Or whole foods and quality core nutrition?

It's your decision.

Calories are Not Created Equal

This is an important distinction. Right now you know exactly how many calories you need to ingest to get you to your weight loss goal. However, *where the calories come from* is also critical. In other words, not all calories are created equal.

Say your daily caloric requirement is 2,000 calories per day. How different is your body going to look if your 2,000 calories come from lean protein and healthy vegetables vs. a couple of Big Macs and fries? The total number of calories is the same...but the results will be vastly different.

When you're fueling your body for weight loss success, your calories come from 5 primary sources:

- ✓ Lean protein
- ✓ Complex carbohydrates

✓ Healthy fats

✓ Fresh fruits

✓ Fibrous vegetables

There's no need to reinvent the wheel. If your calories are coming from these basic sources, you *will* lose weight. You *will* look better. You *will* feel better. And you *will* achieve your goals.

Let's look at each of these items separately...

Lean Protein

Lean protein is the basic building block of any balanced diet. Protein contains amino acids, which are necessary to fuel lean muscle.

I have many friends who are vegetarian or vegan. If this is you, that's great. I think it's a healthy way to go. But I'm not and I don't think I ever will be. I'm going to assume if you're reading this book you're a carnivore like me and you enjoy meat. I will give a couple suggestions if you are someone who is vegan or vegetarian and you're looking for complete sources of protein.

Here are my best sources of protein:

Egg Whites
Turkey (not from Deli)
Lean Ground Turkey Breast
Salmon
Halibut
Orange Roughy
Swordfish

Tuna
Shrimp
Chicken Breasts (Boneless/Skinless)
Buffalo/Bison
Tofu (Vegan)
Black Beans (Vegan)
Nut Butter (Vegan)
Soy/Almond Milk (Vegan)

Complex Carbohydrates

Carbohydrates truly fuel your body. All carbohydrates are eventually broken down into glycogen (the body's stored form of sugar) or glucose (sugar that is ready to be used by the body). The difference between simple and complex carbohydrates is how quickly the body breaks them down and processes them into either sugar or stored energy.

All healthy diets (and especially those focused on sustained weight loss) should focus on *complex carbohydrates*. Low carb/High protein diets are a thing of the past. Most people don't realize this but your body NEEDS carbohydrates to function. Without them, your body doesn't know what to do and it will turn to whatever it can for energy (usually lean muscle tissue). Even your brain needs glucose to function, which is why, if you've ever seen someone on an extremely low carbohydrate diet, they are very irritable and often not as mentally sharp. Their brains are starving for energy.

Here are my best sources of complex carbohydrates:

Wild Rice
Sweet Potatoes
Barley
Steel Cut Oats
Whole Grain Oatmeal
Muesli
Quinoa*
Beans*
Wild Rice
Whole Grain Pasta

*Quinoa and Beans can also be great sources of protein, especially for Vegans

Healthy Fats

Fats are a good thing...assuming you have the right kind. Saturated fats (what you find in butters, sauces, animal fat) are not good. Monounsaturated and Polyunsaturated (mostly found in plants and nuts) are the ones you want to focus on.

Not only are fats good for hair, skin, nails, heart health and lubrication of the joints; they also provide a feeling of satiety, or a feeling of fullness. This is a good thing as I've seen some people attempt an extremely low fat diet and they complain that, no matter how much they eat, it doesn't seem like they ever feel FULL. Healthy fats can help take care of that.

Here are my best sources of healthy fats:

Canola Oil
Extra Virgin Olive Oil

Flaxseed Oil
Nut Butter (also mentioned in protein)
Pecans
Walnuts
Almonds
Pine Nuts
Water Chestnuts
Pistachios
Avocados

Fresh Fruits

Fruits are a simpler form of carbohydrates...the difference being, they are all natural. And the reason they are such a great health and weight loss food is that they provide not only excellent energy; but help hydration (many fruits are more water-based), contain powerful anti-oxidants and anti-inflammatories, as well as many key vitamins and minerals that the body needs. Plus they are refreshing and taste great!

Here are my best sources of fruits:

Bananas
Apples
Grapefruit
Peaches
Strawberries
Blueberries
Raspberries
Blackberries
Pomegranates
Cherries

Pears
Pineapples

Fibrous Vegetables

Vegetables provide fiber that is usually lacking in the American diet. Fiber helps with regularity and helps keep the intestines clean and free from toxic buildup (what I sometimes refer to as "engine sludge"). They also provide essential vitamins, minerals and many of the same anti-oxidant and anti-inflammatory functions that fruits do. Vegetables are usually very low in calories as well...so you can eat them more liberally.

Here are my best sources of vegetables:

Broccoli
Zucchini
Kale
Tomato
Bell Peppers
Asparagus
Carrots
Spinach
Celery
Cucumber
Radishes
Cauliflower
Alfalfa Sprouts
Brussel Sprouts
Cabbage

Foods and Fuels Action Plan

Please keep in mind, this is a non-exhaustive list of healthy foods. If you enjoy something that fits in one of the categories and you KNOW it's healthy, go ahead and continue to have it! I simply listed these foods as a general guide to kick-start your weight loss journey. The next step will be putting together the correct combinations so you can be maximally successful.

First things first, though. Here's your action plan:

1. Go through each list and determine at least 3-5 things that you will eat from each group. If you've never had something, are you willing to experiment with it? The LAST thing I want you to do is to have something you hate, that you know you won't eat and will be miserable if you do...just because you're "supposed to." That's the fastest way to fail on any plan. I tried to give you a comprehensive enough list that you'll have options, and I want you to select things you enjoy AND will help get you where you want to go. So, choose wisely!

Write the foods from each group on your commitment contract. Onward!

CHAPTER 4
PERFECT COMBINATIONS

"In the Formula of Food, 1 + 1 can = 3."

Now that you know what you should be eating, it is time to look at how to put these foods together to get maximum weight loss benefits. The combinations with which you eat foods can have a profound effect on your overall results.

Before going any further, I want to make one point on weight loss. There are LOTS of ways to lose weight. You can lose weight three ways:

- ✓ Lose fat
- ✓ Lose muscle
- ✓ Lose water

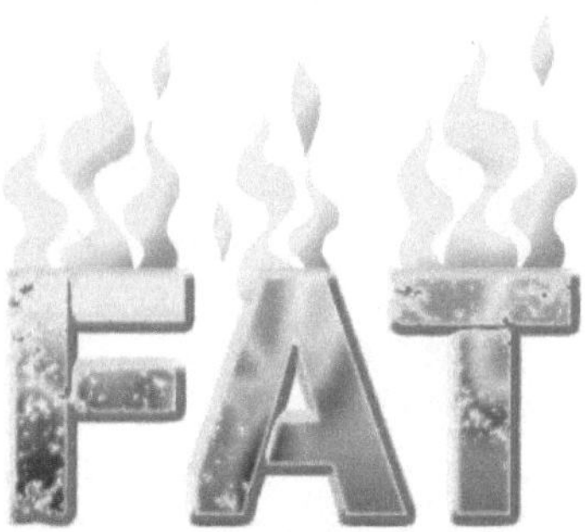

Obviously, this book is about healthy living and losing weight the RIGHT WAY (thus, losing fat) but I do want to touch on the other two points. Losing muscle will likely happen if you restrict your calories too much (below the 1,000 calorie deficit per day from last chapter) or from inadequate protein consumption.

Losing water can happen either from dehydration or, most people don't realize this, it can also happen as a consequence of a high protein diet. High protein diets cause the kidneys to work harder to process protein and excrete waste...thus causing dehydration. A study done at the *University of Connecticut* validates these findings. For people with normal kidney function, it is not that high protein diets are *bad*, they just need to be monitored a bit more carefully, especially when it comes to hydration level.

This is a large contributor to why people lose weight very quickly on high protein diets. Yes, they are losing weight...but it losing water REALLY the right weight that they want to be losing? I'm guessing not.

There are a few basic rules for perfect food combinations that will help you lose weight by *losing fat*. Follow them and you'll be on the fast track to success!

The 'Must Have' Combination

In every meal, you should combine lean protein and complex carbohydrate. This does a couple important things...

First, the *American Journal of Physiology* showed that combining carbohydrate and protein actually facilitates muscle protein synthesis (a good thing). This is *exactly* what you need if you're seeking to change your body SHAPE. You need to hold onto your lean muscle tissue and shed the fat on top of it. Combining protein and carbohydrates together is the best way to ensure this happens.

Second, combining these two macronutrients stabilizes your blood sugar and insulin levels. The *European Journal of Clinical Nutrition* showed combining protein and complex carbohydrates together resulted in greater feelings of energy or lower overall levels of fatigue. Don't we all want that?

Everyone out there reading this probably knows what it feels like to have pure sugar (carbohydrates) in donuts, candy, desserts, etc., and to get the immediate "sugar high," only to come crashing down a short time later. This will happen, to a certain extent, regardless of how complex your carbohydrate source is...but the more complex, the less the spike and the slower the crash. It will still happen but it will be less noticeable. And the best way to make sure it doesn't happen at all is to include lean protein and carbohydrates together at one time.

Below is an example of an ideal meal (please note that a small amount of healthy fat should also be added to this):

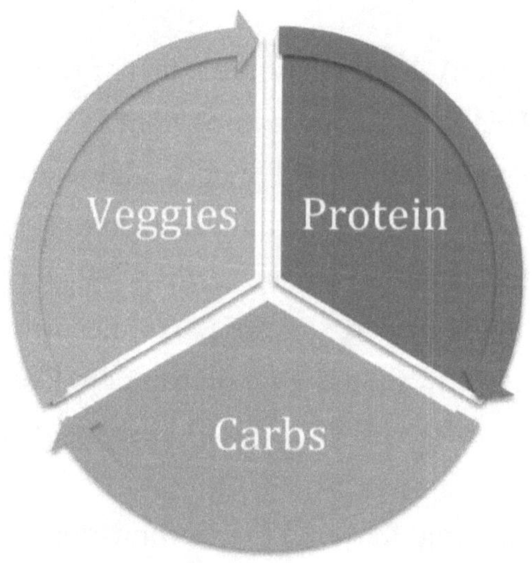

The 'Never Have' Combination

For as facilitative as a protein-carbohydrate combination is for your metabolism, a fat-carbohydrate combination is equally debilitating. Actually, this mostly applies to *saturated fat* combined with carbohydrates.

The reason this is a poor combination is that carbohydrates inherently spike your blood sugar levels, which triggers the release of insulin within your pancreas. This is an obvious problem for Type I diabetics (who don't produce insulin) but I'm actually assuming your body is capable of producing insulin. What happens when you ingest high amount of carbohydrates (especially *simple* carbohydrates) is it puts your body in a state where it wants to use the carbohydrates (sugars) for energy, instead of using stored body fat for energy like we want it to. Adding insult to injury, if we layer on saturated fat on top of these spiked insulin levels there is only one place for it to go – stored body fat. Your body is now working against you!

Now, please remember what we talked about in the first chapter – the all-or-nothing attitude is the death of many weight loss plans. Please don't do that! When I say the "never have combination," I simply mean that you should TRY to never have it...knowing full well that we all, inevitably at some point, will. But it is important to understand these combinations and how having the wrong things together can force us into a nutritional biochemistry where we're actually doing more harm than good. It can easily happen even when we have the best of intentions.

Below is an example of a combination that should be avoided (please note that Fats refer to saturated fats):

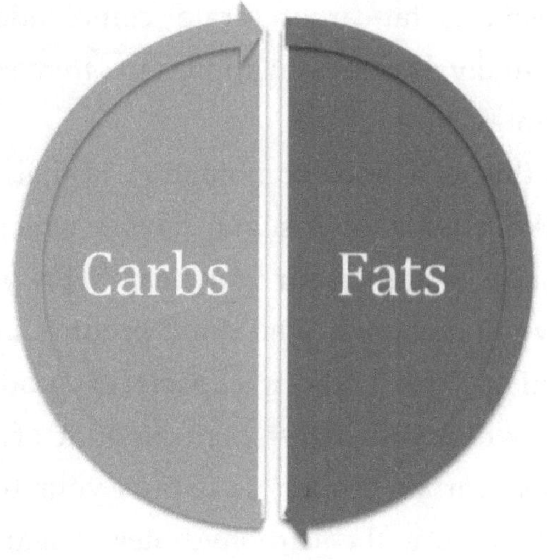

The 'More Often Than Not' Combination

The More Often Than Not Combination is about making sure you have at least 3 servings of vegetables each day and 2-3 servings of fruits. There is a slight difference in how you approach the two.

For vegetables, these can literally be combined with any food throughout the course of the day. Next chapter we will talk about the timing of meals but vegetables can be added to meals or snacks because of their negligible effect on blood sugar or insulin. The role of vegetables is to provide essential vitamins and minerals to the body...as well as a healthy dosage of fiber and a feeling of fullness.

Fruits, on the other hand, need to handled slightly differently. They, too, can be added to any meal but if I were to put it in order of preference, I would steer you towards adding fruits in for breakfast and for snacks. The reason I think it is a great addition for breakfast is because we wake up in a dehydrated state and having water-packed fruits will help with this hydration level. Most fruits can also easily be carried with you in a bag or in a Tupperware container, making them an easy, convenient snack.

Great example of a well-fueled breakfast (again, adding in some healthy fats is fine):

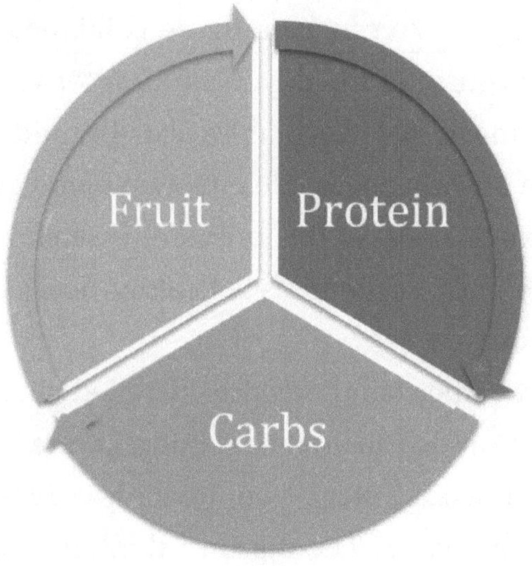

Still aim to have fruits with a lean source of protein, though, as they are a more "simple" form of carbohydrate (depending on which fruit we're talking about) and even though they're also providing essential vitamins and minerals for your body, will affect your insulin levels. So, hitting this combination will keep you losing weight, and most importantly, losing fat.

Perfect Combinations Action Plan

You've already decided which healthy foods from the different groups are your favorites – now it is your turn to decide which ones you are going to combine together.

1. On your commitment contract, play a game of "connect the dots," where you circle food from each group and connect them together in combinations you think you'd like the best. For example, I love to have egg whites in the morning with Steel Cut Oats with a sliced banana mixed into my oatmeal. If I've had a hard workout in the morning I may mix in a bit of Almond Butter or Natural Peanut Butter for some additional healthy fat. But, I would connect the dots for these three (or four) foods. Another alternative to connecting the dots is simply to circle foods in different color markers depending on which ones you'll pair together.

The most important thing is to identify combinations that not only are conducive to weight loss (and fat loss) but also look appealing to you.

CHAPTER 5
NUTRIENT TIMING

"'When' is as Important as 'What' and 'How Much'."

So, to review what we've gone over thus far:

- ✓ You've got the winning attitude
- ✓ You've got the proper amounts
- ✓ You've got the correct foods and fuels
- ✓ You've got the perfect combinations

Whew – that's a great start!

Now it's time to layer in the last thing that *really* matters when it comes to your diet – *nutrient timing*.

You can have everything else correct (and be doing quite well, in fact), but you'll never have an optimal, fully functioning metabolism without nutrient timing. It is like the corner piece that completes the weight loss puzzle. It's THAT important.

It All Starts Here

Growing up, I'd always sleep late and would try to bolt out the door without having breakfast so I could get to school on time. My mom would holler at me, "You know, breakfast is the most important meal of the day!"

I never thought too much about it. I just thought it was something moms say. I could normally have a couple Mountain Dews in the morning and function just fine during school. Or so I thought.

I've come to realize my mom was absolutely right. A proper breakfast can, literally, make or break your day. It sets the tone for everything that follows it. It's really tough to have a bad day after you've had a good breakfast.

First, the word "breakfast" comes from "breaking-a-fast." When you're sleeping you're not only fasting from food; you're also fasting from water. And as we discussed in the *Amounts* chapter, not eating enough will ultimately slow your metabolism over time. So, the fastest way to boost your metabolism in the morning is to have a solid breakfast.

Second, if you're looking for your weight loss to be fat loss, you have to have breakfast. Without it, your body will come up with *some way* to create energy to perform your daily functions and responsibilities. Lack of eating triggers your body to go into starvation mode and if you were paying attention before, this means you'll hold onto stored body fat and actually burn lean muscle tissue for energy. I know, it sounds counter-intuitive, but this is exactly what happens inside of your body.

Third, almost everyone knows what it's like to have wild cravings at night (some know it better than others). Most people think they can beat cravings if they just channel their inner willpower...and they're correct, to a certain extent. But the much larger piece of the puzzle is that being under-caloried (not taking in enough calories) early in the day often leads to hunger and cravings later in the day. Your body gets to a point where it's sick and tired of trying to produce energy from means other than food and it let's you know it. Having a big 'ol breakfast and understanding how this will affect you later in the day is a critical component to metabolism and weight loss.

Here are the standards you need to meet for breakfast if you want to be successful. No BS here. Please meet them or you *will not* lose weight.

- ✓ 20 grams of protein within 30 minutes of waking up
- ✓ Minimum of 200 calories; Maximum of 600 calories.
- ✓ 16-20 ounces of water*

Include fruit for further hydration.

Two quick things to mention:

If you're having foods from a package, you can pretty easily eyeball it and see whether it adds up to 20 grams of protein. Some great sources to make sure you're meeting your minimum amounts of protein are Greek yogurt, about 4 egg whites or ¾ cup of cottage cheese. Of course, there are many great meal replacement shakes and bars available, and if you are choosing another source of lean protein, following the "palm of your hand" guide to portion sizing will put you at roughly 20 grams.

Also, if you are someone who exercises FIRST thing in the morning (I hope you are!), you do not *have to* eat beforehand...unless you find that you'll get lightheaded during your workout if you don't. Instead, perform your workout but make sure to have your breakfast within *30 minutes of completion* of your workout. This will not only help you rebuild and recover from the exercise; it will trigger the same metabolic response for the day.

Nutrient Frequency

I always tell my clients to be grazers, not bingers. Basically, this means to have small meals and snacks, frequently, throughout the course of the day. Doing this sets your metabolism up to hold onto lean muscle tissue and shed the fat on top of it, which is EXACTLY what you want if you're looking to lose weight and change the shape of your body in the process.

The standard for nutrient frequency is to eat every 3-4 hours with the combination of protein and carbohydrate (ideal) or healthy fats and carbohydrate (secondary). For most people, their eating schedule would look something like this:

Breakfast (7am) > Mid-Morning Snack (9:30am) > Lunch (12:30pm) > Mid-Afternoon Snack (3:30pm) > Dinner (7pm)

Of course, your times may differ somewhat from these but you get the idea. Putting quality nutrients into your body every 3-4 hours is ESSENTIAL to your program.

Sometimes people worry about not being hungry every 3-4 hours, which is where portion sizing comes in. Your meals or snacks should not contain any more than 600 calories at any one sitting (and this would only be for someone who is very active). For most people, the 3 "square" meals of breakfast, lunch and dinner would be between 400-500 calories and snacks would be 200-300 calories. This will put you somewhere around 1500-2500 total calories for the day and this is where the great majority of people looking to lose weight (the *healthy way*) need to be.

I often use the analogy of a fire to simulate nutrient timing. When you have consistent nutrient frequency, you have a steady flame always burning on your fire. THAT'S what you want! You don't want the flame to burn out and you have to start it up again. You also don't want to pour so much wood on the fire (food) that your fire burns out of control (what happens when we eat too much).

Now, I get it – life is going to get in the way sometimes. These things happen. Your kids will have an emergency or you'll have a fire you have to put out at work. Just go with it and move on. Start fresh the next day. But, I will tell you this – the greatest cause of people not eating every 3-4 hours is lack of planning. Plain and simple. If you leave it up to chance and say, "I'll eat when I have a break in my day," it'll never happen. You may be able to get away with it here or there but it's not sustainable. We're all too busy and our schedules will get in the way.

To have nutrient frequency, planning becomes doubly important. When you go to bed at night you should have a good idea what you'll be eating the next day. Of course, if you happen to be going out for lunch or dinner, I don't *expect* you to know exactly what you're going to order...but you SHOULD know when those meals are going to happen. Everything else should be planned for. If you don't do this simple thing, meals are going to be missed, metabolisms are going to be slowed, and results are going to be a lot harder to come by.

The Nighttime Taper

Most people are more active earlier in the day than they are later. When you get to dinnertime (and certainly, after), your combinations should be shifted more towards protein and less towards carbohydrates.

Why? It comes back to a simple principle that your body is going to store *anything* in excess as body fat. Protein, fats, carbohydrates – it doesn't matter. Have too much of it and your body will store it. And with diminished activity later in the day, our bodies don't require the same amount of carbohydrates as it does earlier. It doesn't need the same type of fuel to sustain function.

This doesn't mean you have to steer totally away from carbohydrates. A piece of fruit or a small amount of complex carbohydrates is fine. But too many carbohydrates (especially complex ones) are unnecessary. Better to shift the ratios towards protein for lean tissue (ideal) or a small amount of healthy fats for internal function (secondary).

Great examples of this could be a protein shake (usually whey or a plant-based protein) mixed with Almond Milk or a piece of fruit and a handful of almonds. A protein bar that is low in sugar could also be an excellent choice.

Nutrient Timing Action Plan

To reiterate, the most critical part of nutrient timing is planning. It's knowing *when* you're going to eat *what*. Having a sound plan of action will go a long ways to ensuring your weight loss success.

1. Simple question – what is your favorite breakfast? Please don't say donuts – we're talking about foods that fall within these weight loss guidelines! Decide what a standard, healthy breakfast would look like for you and write it on your commitment contract (feel free to go back to Foods and Fuels if you need a refresher on some healthy choices). There are spaces to write in 3 different breakfasts so if you think you'll get bored having the same thing day after day, feel free to come up with more than one. Start the day out right!

2. Weekdays are the most difficult time for most people to adhere to the schedule of eating every 3-4 hours. It's this way for almost everyone. So, your first step is to determine WHEN you're going to be eating during your day throughout the course of a regular week. Write this on your commitment contract.

I don't mean to keep drilling on this point but you HAVE TO know when you'll be eating. When you're writing your times on your commitment contract, don't say you'll eat something at 9:30am if you typically have work meetings during this time and you know you can't eat. Look at your schedule and put some constructive thought into it. When can you legitimately make it happen so it is realistic with your work/lifestyle and also with the nutrient timing guidelines.

CHAPTER 6
EXERCISE TO BOOST METABOLISM

"Your Metabolism is like a Furnace. Turn Yours Up!"

By now you understand that you have to create a caloric deficit to lose weight. It's the one non-negotiable aspect of weight. It cannot happen any other way.

Up to this point all the focus has been on creating this caloric deficit through nutrition but there is another equally qualified way to do this – exercise.

Most people think of exercise and grimace...especially if you've failed on diets or weight loss plans in the past. They think of exercise as running on the hamster wheel or boringly spinning away on the elliptical, counting down the seconds until you can stop.

It doesn't have to be that way.

Trust me – you CAN find a way to make exercise fun, burn calories and create the necessary deficit you need to. Triple win! You can do this because the beautiful thing about exercise nowadays is there are many small, niche classes going on everywhere. All you have to do is look around and you'll find something that you not only find interesting but also beneficial to your weight loss.

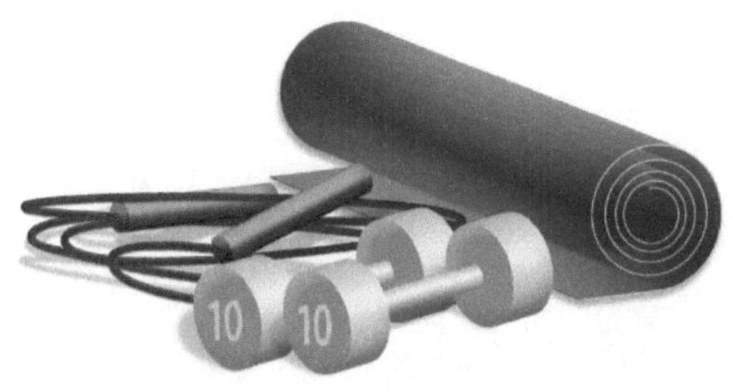

Some examples (I can't guarantee these are going on in your area but, yes, these all are real world classes):

- ✓ Spinning
- ✓ Pilates
- ✓ Pole dancing
- ✓ Step class
- ✓ Barre
- ✓ Crossfit
- ✓ Core Power Yoga
- ✓ Water aerobics
- ✓ Running/Walking clubs
- ✓ Zumba
- ✓ Bootcamp

This is actually only a short list of classes off the top of my head. I've tried almost all of them (um, except pole dancing) and they all bring a unique flavor and challenges. You simply have to be willing to step outside of your comfort zone and give them a shot. I guarantee if you do this and give it an honest chance, you will find something that works for you.

However, if you are someone who is anti-classes or working out in groups, I'm going to clearly lay out some of the general guidelines regarding exercise and what you need to do to make it the most beneficial for weight loss. The big benefit to working out in classes is accountability (discussed more later), social support and motivation, but you do not get an individual, customized workout based on what you NEED. These guidelines will help you attack the latter and provide a good starting point for when you are looking for the right type of class to fit your goals.

The Truth About Exercise

Your BMR accounts for 60-75% of the calories you burn every day. The number of calories your body burns at rest is critical to your weight loss and the more you can "stoke" your metabolic fire, the better chance you have at succeeding.

I've worked with hundreds of clients on weight loss and here's the harsh truth - you can exercise until you're blue in the face, but if you're not putting good quality core nutrition into your mouth, you'll *never* see the weight loss results you want to. That's the truth...and that's the reason why this book has spent so much time discussing nutrition. Food has to be the foundational layer in which everything else is layered on top of it.

In reality, it's probably an 80/20 split, where 80% of your results will come from nutrition and 20% from exercise.

All that being said, exercise will absolutely *impact* your weight loss results. You cannot do it with exercise alone but you certainly can accelerate it by adding in quality exercise. The TYPE of exercise will have a dramatic effect on your body shape and composition and, of course, there are the *substantial* health benefits that come from exercise. So, by no means am I telling you to not worry about exercise. I love everything about exercise. I just want to make sure we're on the same page about what really matters *most* when it comes to losing weight.

The Best Type of Exercise to Burn Calories

In terms of bang for your buck, strength training is the best form of exercise you can do. You have three basic choices when it comes to exercise (and each of these are fine based on your personality and what you like) – take an exercise class, do a home-based DVD program or create your own workout. The rest of this chapter will deal mainly with creating your own workout.

For years, I heard that one pound of muscle burns 40-50 calories at rest, whereas one pound of fat only burns 2-3 calories at rest. Recent studies are starting to challenge whether the discrepancy is actually *that* great, but regardless, muscle burns A LOT more calories than fat. And because your BMR accounts for such a high percentage of your daily caloric expenditure, it makes sense to add lean muscle to your body. This ensures that your metabolism is maximally efficient at rest.

Strength training is essential for creating your best body *shape* as well. For people who do not perform any strength training but have gone on a diet (you may know some of these people), sometimes they are able to lose weight but they don't necessarily *look* any smaller. This is because they are still the same shape they were before...there's just less of them.

Sometimes, when I discuss strength training, people fear getting "bulky" (women especially). This will not happen. In the case of females, the extreme majority is incapable of putting on muscle mass because they don't secrete the necessary hormones (testosterone, mostly). And many people don't realize that strength training will actually make you look SMALLER because muscle is more dense than fat...meaning it takes us less space. This is a great thing.

The last big benefit from strength training comes from retaining lean muscle as we age. Most studies say we will start losing muscle after the age of 25 (with the most significant losses happening after age 50) if we don't do something to prevent it. That's exactly what strength training does – it not only helps you keep your lean muscle, which in turn, keeps your body strong and resistance to the general aches and pains and pulled muscles that happen more easily as we age.

Now you understand why strength training is important, so if you're picking an exercise class to start attending, I'd highly recommend picking one that incorporates strength training. And just note that this doesn't have to mean you're lifting heavy weights – strength training can also comes in the form of supporting your own bodyweight, which is common in classes like Yoga, Pilates and Barre.

If you are putting together a strength-training program for yourself, here are the basic "Do This, Not That" guidelines:

Do This: Work big muscle groups
Not That: Work small muscle groups

The biggest muscle groups in the body are the legs (hamstrings, thighs and butt), chest, back and shoulders. When you work these muscle groups, your body has to work harder, you burn more calories and you see greater results. These big muscle groups should be the backbone of any strength-training program.

Smaller muscle groups include arms, calves and abs. When you work these muscle groups your body doesn't have to work as hard and you burn less calories. I'm not saying you need to totally leave the muscles alone and never touch them – I am simply saying to make sure you *prioritize* working big muscle groups first to see the greatest benefit.

Here are my favorite exercises for the big muscle groups:

Chest
- ✓ Pushups
- ✓ Dips or Assisted Dips

Back
- ✓ Lat Pull
- ✓ Pullups or Assisted Pullups

Shoulders
- ✓ Shoulder Press
- ✓ Dumbbell Lateral Raise

Thighs
- ✓ Squats

Hamstrings
- ✓ Deadlifts

Butt
- ✓ Step Ups
- ✓ Lunges

Do This: Compound exercises
Not That: Simple exercises

Compound exercises are ones where you're working multiple muscle groups at once. The exercises burn more calories than simple exercises because you're working more muscles at once (they'll be more difficult, but you get more benefit). For the newer exerciser, this could be a squat, lunge or step up. For the advanced exerciser, this could be a squat with a row, lunge with a bicep curl or step up with a shoulder press. Simple exercises would be a leg extension, hamstring curl or calf raise. Keep these to a minimum.

Do This: Exercises where you support your own bodyweight
Not That: Exercises where you're on a machine

For the most part, exercises where you're locked into a machine should be left alone. Normally, these machines have you locked into a fixed plane of motion (the first downfall), have you sitting down (the second downfall) and you do not have you engaging any of your secondary "stabilizer" muscles like you would need to if you were standing up and supporting your own bodyweight (the third downfall).

I do realize, not every exercise can be done standing up. But let's say you're doing a chest press with dumbbells – you'd be much better off doing them on a stability ball than you would on a machine. Again, it simply comes down to the number of calories you're burning and the bang for your buck you're getting out of exercise.

Do This: Circuit training with very short rest periods
Not That: Anything with longer rest periods

When I walk into a gym these days I look around and see half the people playing with the iPods. Why? Queue up your playlist before you start and let it run through your entire workout – what needs to be changed? For most people, this is just a stall tactic.

Keep your rest periods VERY short when you're strength training, preferably as short as 30-45 seconds. Most people would call this "circuit training," which traditionally means that you bounce from one exercise to the next with very little rest in between.

If you've never done strength training like this before, it takes some getting used to. First, 30-45 seconds goes by in the blink of an eye. Second, it requires some planning on how and where you're going to perform the exercises to make sure able to do them without taking a longer rest. Third, you're probably going to be breathing heavy throughout, which leads to the greatest benefit of circuit training – it keeps your heart rate elevated the entire time and, again, helps you to burn the most calories (do you notice a pattern forming here?).

If you're interested in sample workout programs please visit the **OutperformTheNorm.com/books** for free access.

Maximizing Your Exercise

All of health, fitness and weight loss (and LIFE, for that matter) are based on creating *Progressive Overload*. Your body is a phenomenally adaptive machine and this terms states that by progressively overloading your body with greater intensities, it will positively adapt and grow stronger (and thus, lose weight). When I was full-time personal training, every single thing we did was based around this simple concept.

HOW you create the progressive overload is a different thing altogether. The next chapter is going to be geared towards the measurement of what you're doing and what that's so important.

But, for now, we need to look at progressive overload in terms of making sure you're challenging yourself to do a little and to be a little better, each day. Isn't it funny how philosophies for weight loss also seem like winning strategies for life?

Most people think that duration (how *long* you work out) is the primary factor in creating progressive overload. It's not. Longer isn't always better. Assuming your rest periods are staying constant at 30-45 seconds between exercises, these are some of the other ways you could create progressive overload in strength training:

- ✓ Lift heavier weights
- ✓ Perform more repetitions (the number of times you do an exercise consecutively)
- ✓ Perform more sets (the number of times you repeat the repetition cycle)
- ✓ Perform more exercises (the total number of different exercises you're doing)
- ✓ Frequency of strength training (how many days per week you're exercising)

None of these are bad, but my advice is to keep the focus on creating progressive overload through #1 and #2. The last 3 would have the biggest impact on duration and your time commitment exercising and I try to respect the fact that we're ALL busy people. This is the reason that I sound like a broken record and I keep coming back to getting the best results in the shortest times.

Focusing on #2, 20-25 repetitions is plenty...any more than that and you're probably not challenging yourself enough, in which case, you shift to #1, where you increase the amount of weight you're lifting. If you are doing bodyweight exercises, you can challenge yourself through different positions and angles. Think of doing a pushup with hands on the table and feet on the floor (easier) versus doing a standard pushup (more difficult).

You're probably wondering if I'm ever going to talk about cardiovascular exercise. I would have mentioned it earlier but, in terms of bang for your buck, you'll actually get more out of a quality strength training session (from a metabolism standpoint) than you will from cardiovascular exercise. It is not that cardiovascular exercise is *bad* (c'mon, you're talking to someone who loves it!) – I'm just trying to make you maximally efficient with your time.

Cardiovascular exercise follows the same exact progressive overload principles of strength training. Are longer durations of cardiovascular exercise better than shorter durations? Sure. But I would still focus on #1 and #2 from above...the only difference being, #1 means you're going faster or have more resistance on whatever type of cardiovascular equipment you're using. #2 would be if you're performing an interval program. The intervals would not need to be longer than 1 minute in duration and once you get to a point where you are doing 10 of them (regardless of your method of cardiovascular exercise), you should go back to #1 and start increasing the intensity of the interval. The rest periods are similar to strength training and by constantly flip-flopping between #1 and #2 you will be ensured of creating progressive overload.

A great tool to use to gauge your cardiovascular exercise can be a heart rate monitor, which indicates how hard your heart is working during exercise. Please see the Bonus section towards the end of the book for more details.

As a guide, here are my best forms of cardiovascular exercise:

(most beneficial to least beneficial)

- ✓ Treadmill
- ✓ Stair stepper
- ✓ Rowing machine
- ✓ Upright bike
- ✓ Recumbent bike
- ✓ Hand cycle

Almost every health club will have these selections.

Exercise Action Plan

Planning goes into exercise as much, if not more, than it does nutrition. You HAVE TO eat, so a lot of proper nutrition is simply having the right things available and putting them into your mouth rather than the wrong things. But you do not have to exercise and, until you're at a place where exercise has been fully ingrained as a habit, you will probably allow other things to trump your exercise if they come up. I don't say that derogatorily—I say it because I've seen it before.

1. On your commitment contract, write down the type of exercise you're going to perform, where you're going to do it and how often you're going to make it happen. This is the starting point to adhering to any exercise program.

2. Determine WHEN you will exercise. If, at all possible, do it first thing in the morning. Like breakfast, I'm a big believer in starting the day out right and when you start it out with a healthy does of exercise to stoke your metabolism, it's tough to have a bad day after that. On your commitment contract, write the time you are most likely to exercise.

Then, if you *really* want to be successful, take out your phone and open up the calendar (or paper calendar, if that's how you roll) and SCHEDULE it into your day like you would any other meeting. Put it as a meeting of high importance and do your very best to not let anything interrupt it. You'd be surprised how things fit into other areas of your day when you make this commitment and you do not alter it.

CHAPTER 7
MEASURING PROGRESS

"Focus on Progress, NOT Perfection."

I'm a big believer that progress leads to happiness and fulfillment. Everyone likes to know that they're doing the *right* thing; that they're getting *better* at something. It's human nature to want to be good at the things we do.

From a health and fitness perspective, I don't believe we're ever "maintaining." Our health is always either progressing or regressing. It's never staying exactly the same.

Now, from a weight loss perspective, you may be questioning what I'm talking about, thinking that I want you to continue losing weight for the rest of your life or you're not making progress? Not at all. See – every single person out there reading this book right now is aging (so is the person who is writing it!) and because we have a tendency to lose lean muscle as we age, which slows our metabolism, it takes an equal or greater amount of work just to *stay where we are.*

So, to me, maintaining your weight can still be looked at as making progress. Hopefully that makes sense.

Progress is also an exceptional motivator. Think of taking a long road trip in your car to a foreign destination. Your GPS will always give you an estimated time of arrival, right? Sometimes, at the beginning, it may seem that the destination will never be reached but as you get closer and closer to it, momentum and motivation grow. You get excited for your arrival.

Not looking at progress is likely blinding driving in a general direction, with no real idea when you'll ever arrive at your destination. At times, you're not even sure whether you're lost or on the right track. If this happens enough times, you throw in the towel altogether and quit, saying "that just didn't work for me."

Measuring progress let's you know that what you're doing is WORKING.

What Gets Measured Gets Mastered

If you ask any successful businessperson about their numbers, they're going to know them backwards and forwards. They'll know revenue, profit, expenses, trends, etc. Why? What gets measured gets mastered.

I often tell people, you CANNOT evaluate what you cannot measure. You don't know if what you're doing is working or whether you're spinning your wheels. Measurement not only lets you know if you're making progress, it also provides feedback and learning if you're not doing the right thing.

Of the successful people I've seen lose weight, they were all methodical about measuring their results. It didn't mean they were always happy with the measurements or with the results they saw...but they were committed to them nonetheless.

Measuring Progress Action Plan

There are four basic areas to look at measurements:

- ✓ Biomarkers
- ✓ Food
- ✓ Hydration
- ✓ Exercise

Biomarkers

Biomarkers could theoretically be everything from your internal blood chemistries to your hormone levels. But the primary biomarkers we're looking at in this case are weight, body composition and girth measurements (inches). Each of these tell a slightly different story. We've already discussed how weight can come from losing fat, losing water or losing muscle, and this is where body composition and girth measurements help determine that what you're losing is, indeed, the right stuff (losing fat).

Taking girth measurements is relatively simple – all you need is a tape measure (like you would use for sewing). To have your body composition checked, your best bet is probably to ask a fitness professional at your health club. If you do not belong to a health club, ask a doctor or medical professional. They will be able to point you in the right direction.

I will not tell you that you have to do all of them but I WILL tell you that the more of them you do, the better chances you'll have for success. At the bare minimum, you should do either body composition or girth measurements. Record these on your commitment contract.

As far as frequency, body composition and girth measurements should not be checked any more than once per week. I recommend weighing yourself every other day to keep your goal in the forefront of your mind. Just please remember that subtle shifts in weight can happen due to retaining water, monthly cycles, sodium consumption, etc. You should not expect that your weight is ALWAYS going to be lower every time you weigh yourself. Focus on the general *trend* of weight loss and you will be successful.

Food

For food, we're strictly talking about recording and measuring your food. Let me say this – the simplest way to do it is through an app on your phone. My personal favorites are *Lose It* and *My Fitness Pal*. Either one will allow the simple tracking of your daily food and caloric intake.

If you're someone who does not do apps, you should still write down all the foods you're eating (access the tracker at **OutperformTheNorm.com/books**, if you need one). I do not expect you to write down calories for every single food you eat. That would be *seriously* time consuming. I do think it's a good idea to write down the foods just for the reflection of your eating habits and to be cognizant of what you're actually putting in your mouth. Studies have actually shown that people who write their foods down are more successful on weight loss plans.

Hydration

This one is simple – write down the number of ounces of water you're drinking each day, make a note in your phone or record it in your app. ONLY water and naturally flavored water counts. Any other sodas, coffees, teas, etc., do not count towards your total daily water intake.

Exercise

Again, this is where the apps have changed the game in terms of measuring and recording your exercise. The same apps mentioned before will record everything you're doing from an exercise standpoint. If you're someone who doesn't do apps, make a notation in your calendar, either paper or on your phone. Be sure to label the type of exercise you did and the total exercise time (for cardiovascular exercise, especially).

CHAPTER 8

ACCOUNTABILITY AND SUPPORT

"We Were Put on this Planet to Pull Other People Up."

Having a support system is a necessary component for successful weight loss. We talked about it in the first chapter with *Resiliency*. Things are NOT always going to be easy in your journey to lose weight. In fact, there will probably be times where it feels damn near impossible. You'll be frustrated because life is getting in the way (it happens), the scale isn't moving (it also happens) and you feel like giving up (don't let it happen). This is where you need a support system the most.

For years, a support system has been the backbone of many successful programs (think of drug and alcohol rehab). Now, I'm not saying you have to join a local group, where you stand up in front of the room as say, "Hi, my name is Jane and I have a weight problem." That might not be your personality. But I am telling you that it's critical to have someone there to support you when times get tough and you need it the most.

Even the most determined, confident people get beat up. And sometimes we need someone to believe in us when it's difficult for us to believe in ourselves.

Determining YOUR Best Support System

Everybody needs a support system but how you would like to be supported is based on your individual personality. People typically fall into one of two categories:

Public Support

If you are an extravert, this choice is probably for you. The best thing you can do is to tell everyone what you're doing and join a group of like-minded people with the same goal of weight loss. Many health clubs have ongoing weight loss programs and classes going on constantly. Join one so you can be supported.

Other means of public support would be to ask family, friends and co-workers to be there and support you when the times get tough.

Private Support

This is the choice for introverts. The beauty of technology is that there are many readily accessible forums and groups for people who are looking for weight loss. The difference here being, you can be a part of these groups and still remain relatively anonymous. You can stand on the outside looking in and be a part of a community, without feeling like you need to social with other people (if that's not your thing) and be front and center.

Regardless of which one you choose, please understand that a support system is a crucial and *necessary* component to your weight loss success. Very few (if any) people do it alone. Having some type of support system (public or private) lets you be a part of something and feel like you're not alone in your journey.

Being Accountable

We ALL need to be held accountable from time to time. Even the most successful people I've met (in every area of life) need accountability. It keeps them on task, keeps them from wavering and keeps them doing exactly what they have initially set out to do.

An accountability partner for weight loss does the same exact thing.

Who is going to hold you accountable in this journey? It could be a group, a coach, a friend or a family member. It really doesn't matter. What matters is that, instead of being a support system to pull you up if you're feeling down, an accountability partner is more for making sure you're doing the *right things*. They're kind of like the teacher making sure you're doing your homework.

I'm personally a fan of screaming out your goals loud and clear, for the world to hear, so everyone knows you're all in. When you do that, you can't go back. You either do it or you face the fear of everyone knowing you did not do what you set out to do...which, in turn, acts as a powerful motivator for action. But I understand this isn't for everybody.

Believe it or not, accountability can actually come from an app or writing things into a calendar or journal as well. You know you are accountable to SOMETHING. At the end of the day, I still think it's best to have a *person* holding you accountable but measuring and logging all your biomarkers, food, hydration and exercise data, and having to look at it staring back at you, is certainly better than nothing.

Accountability Action Plan

1. What will be your Support System? Will you function the best with a public or private support system? Write what your support system will be on your commitment contract.

2. Who will be your accountability partner? Do you have someone who could join you in your weight loss journey? When you think of this person, make sure they're someone who is going to be ok with holding you accountable, meaning they won't be afraid to "politely scold" you if you're not doing the things you said you were going to do. We all need to be told this every now and then...which is why coaching has become such a popular profession. We perform better when we know someone is watching us.

If you do not have a person and you'd prefer to be held accountable in another way, that's ok (this should be the last resort, though). Whatever your method of accountability, please write it on your commitment contract.

Conclusion

If you've made it this far there's nothing left to say. There's only left to DO.

I've seen a lot of people be successful with weight loss...and keep it off. I've also seen people try and try and try and try and never truly succeed. So, I'll go back to where I started - it all comes down to *attitude*. Like anything in life, you're the variable. And the people I've seen who have not been successful have simply not had the proper attitude, level of disgust, commitment, plan and resiliency to make a profound, lasting change that will ultimately improve their life.

Every week (literally) there's a new diet book coming out: Atkins, Keto, South Beach, Zone, FAST, Hormone, Doctor's, Paleo, Gluten-free, Shred, Military, 3-2-1—and these are only the tip of the iceberg.

Are some of these better than others? Sure. But I'll let you in on a little tip – lots of things WORK. But NOTHING will *ever* work if you don't stick to it. Every single thing in life that is worthwhile requires a commitment and a sacrifice, and with this comes value. Think about the things you truly *value* in your life – did they come easy? I bet not. You had to *work* for them. With hard work comes value and appreciation of the journey.

It is my hope that you'll take the strategies in this book and apply them consistently, and immediately, to lose weight so you look the way you want to look and feel the way you want to feel.

You deserve THAT. All of these principles are surprisingly simple, yet grounded in sound scientific rationale. They've worked for others. Follow them and they *will* work for you.

Remember, you're the variable. Go out and make it happen.

Best of Life and Keep Outperforming,
Scott

BONUSES

FREE Gift

If you'd like to go a little further please accept this gift...

100% Absolutely Free

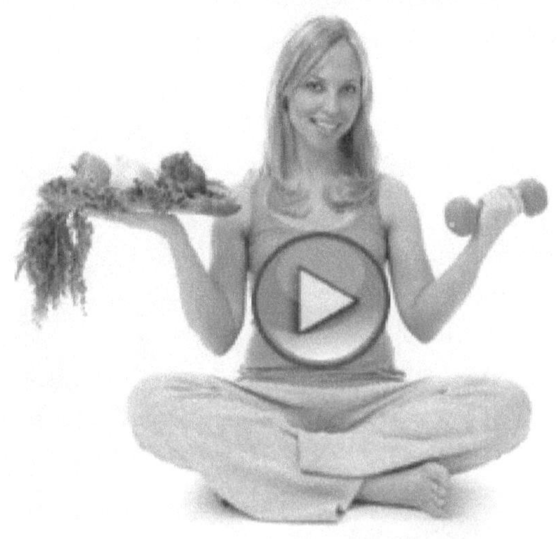

The Exclusive Create LEAN Webinar

Looking the way you want to look and feeling the way you want to feel aren't things that randomly happen. They are things you CREATE. And once it is created, it's a lot easier to maintain it. But if you've never mastered the principles of what it takes to Create LEAN, then it's likely leading to on-and-off cravings, weight fluctuation, fad diets and frustrations.

This is a **no-cost**, high value webinar from the Create LEAN series that will show you the advanced strategies I've successfully used to help clients get lean for years (and help myself!). Please join me…it'll be worth your while.

OutperformTheNorm.com/books

I'll "see" you there.

Scott

Sample Strength Training Program

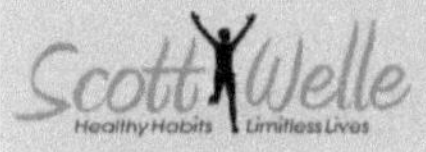
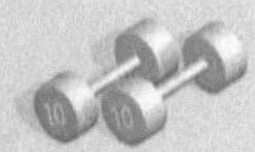

1. Step Lunge

Sets	Reps	Weight	Notes
1	30	X	15 on each side
2	30	X	15 on each side
3	30	X	15 on each side

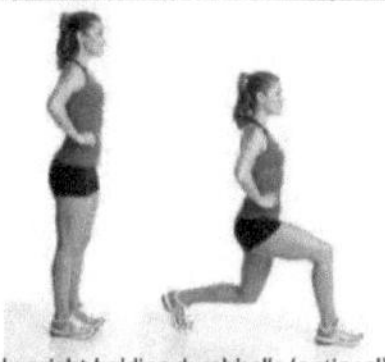

1 – Stand upright holding dumbbells (optional) by your sides with arms straight.

2 – Take a step forward, dropping your back knee down and leaning your torso slightly forward with your weight on your front leg.

3 – Push off your front foot to return to start position.

2. Ball Dumbbell Chest Press

Sets	Reps	Weight	Notes
1	15		
2	15		
3	15		

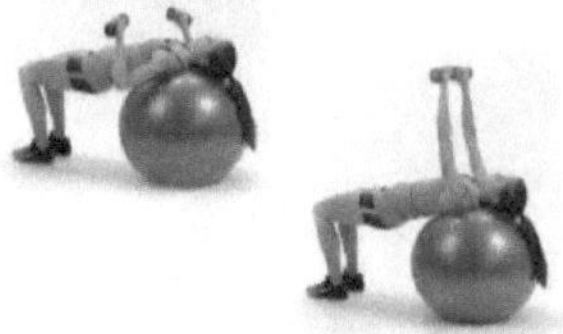

1 - Lie with your upper back on the ball holding dumbbells at shoulder level, elbows bent.

2 - Press the dumbbells up until your arms are straight over your chest.

3 - Lower the dumbbells back to shoulder level, keeping your hips in line with your shoulders.

3. Step Up

Sets	Reps	Weight	Notes
1	20		10 on each side
2	20		10 on each side
3	20		10 on each side

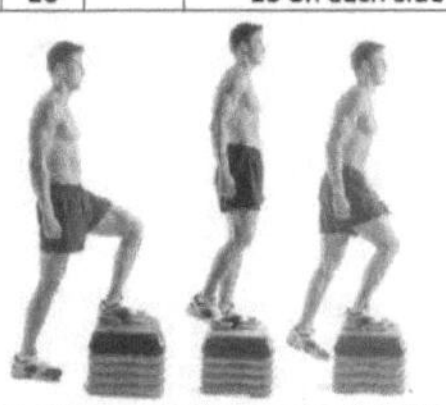

1 - Stand upright with one foot on a bench, holding dumbbells (optional) by your sides with your arms straight.

2 - Step up onto the bench, pushing down on your front foot.

3 - Step down off the bench onto the back foot and repeat.

4. Seated Cable Row

Sets	Reps	Weight	Notes
1	12		
2	12		
3	12		

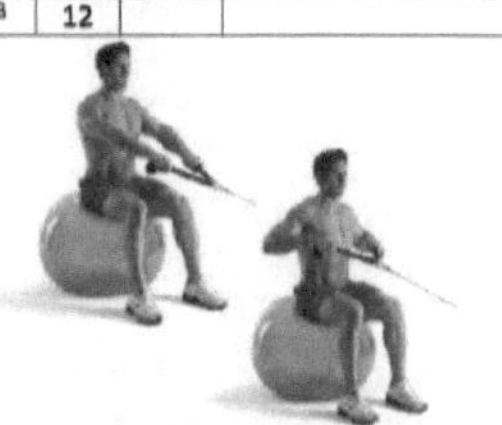

1 - Sit on a ball or a bench holding the handles with your arms straight using the close grip with your palms facing in and your chest against the pad.

2 - Pull the handles straight in to your chest, bending at the elbows.

3 - Straighten your arms, returning to the start position.

OutperformTheNorm.com/books

Monitoring Intensity by Heart Rate

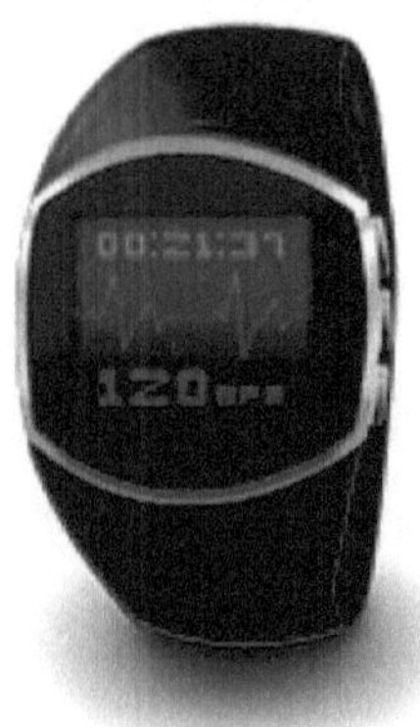

The heart is the core of your body's power plant. It is the strongest muscle in your body. For as long as you are alive, your heart never stops beating. As you rest, move, and exercise, your heart constantly self-regulates its action to provide your muscles and organs with the energy they need. Your heart rate is variable and complex, especially during stressful activity.

To understand your body's fitness, you need to be aware of what your heart is doing from moment to moment. The heart rate is the efficiency rating of the entire body. As your fitness improves, your heart rate improves with it. This is where a Heart Rate Monitor comes in.

Here are just a few of the powerful benefits of using a Heart Rate Monitor:

- ✓ Exercise becomes more time-efficient and safe
- ✓ Fitness programs can be more easily personalized and made fun
- ✓ Workout intensity can be measured simply and reliably
- ✓ Results become apparent that might otherwise not be seen
- ✓ Goals are more easily set and reached
- ✓ Progress toward fitness is easily tracked
- ✓ Motivation to improve increases
- ✓ Confidence is bolstered and reinforced
- ✓ Knowledge replaces guesswork

A Heart Rate Monitor is not just for structured exercise. It can help turn any activity into a workout.

Overcoming Obstacles and Reaching Fitness

Statistics show that over 70% of the people who start an exercise program will quit within the first six months and many within the first few weeks. What makes it so hard for individuals to stick with an exercise program? Why do they give up so quickly?

Most people start an exercise program with a specific goal or need in mind. That is the driving force or motivation behind their desire to exercise. However, many people run into common obstacles that cause them to lose sight of these goals, and so they begin to lose their motivation to keep going.

Fortunately, a heart rate monitor can provide the solution to many of the obstacles that stand in the way of your success in an exercise program!

One challenge lies in understanding the connection between heart rate and fitness. If your heart rate is too low during exercise, your body reaps little or no benefits. This means you are not likely to see the results you want, like weight loss or increased endurance. On the other hand, if your heart rate is too high during exercise, you may tire too quickly and become frustrated. You even run the risk of injury. In either case, you are likely to quit exercising because you are not getting the results you want. A Heart Rate Monitor assures you that you are in the right zone for the workout you're doing.

Heart Rate Monitoring

Why use a heart rate monitor?

Another problem is in measuring the most useful heart rate. Different techniques measure different pulses, and the techniques required to take the correct pulse accurately can be tricky or intimidating. Even at best, a finger on the right pulse can only give a ballpark of the most valuable heart rate for fitness measurement, which is electrical. A Heart Rate Monitor is easy to put on and use, and gives consistent results.

Without a Heart Rate Monitor, it can be difficult to track your progress. The advantage is obvious to exercising with a device that can record your heart rate over time, perform complex calculations for you, and provide reliability in measurements. The overall trend of fitness becomes easy to see. Your fitness knowledge is no longer confined to counting between heartbeats; with a Heart rate Monitor keeping track, that knowledge skyrockets to a total life perspective.

Finally, it can be frustrating to begin an exercise program when the apparent results seem so far down the road. It takes four to six weeks of consistent exercise before you begin to see any external changes to your body. Yet, internal improvements begin to take place immediately although you can't see them. A Heart Rate Monitor can reveal that the inside is changing -- it is reassuring to know that the outside can't be too far behind.

So if you want to have effective workouts, maximize your exercise experience, be motivated by seeing real changes and be able to track those changes, then a heart rate monitor is the best tool for the job.

Who should use an HRM?

Anyone who wants to:

- Burn more calories in the same amount of time
- Avoid guessing their work intensity
- Increase motivation to exercise
- Understand the numbers that make exercise valuable and create accountability
- Know data such as calories burned, average HR, time in target zone, etc.
- Have different workout types in order to make exercise interesting (some would even call it FUN!)

- ✓ Increase cardiovascular conditioning and reduce chance of cardiovascular disease
- ✓ Lower their resting heart rate
- ✓ Increase their metabolism and overall body efficiency
- ✓ Provide the right mixes of aerobic (longer time spent) and anaerobic (higher intensity) exercise to increase AT and VO2 Max
- ✓ Avoid over-training

Why use a heart rate monitor?

Why can't I just take my own heart rate by putting my finger on my neck or wrist?

It has been found that people who used this method -- called the palpitation method -- found that their palpated rates were 13 beats per minute (bpm) less than electronic rates following the 1-mile walk and 17 bpm less following the 1-mile jog. Thirteen beats per minute can take you into an entirely different exercise intensity than what you had originally intended.

Why can't I just hold on to the handles on the exercise machines and get my heart rate there?

Holding on to the pulse meters while exercising is not advised. You cannot get a moment-to- moment reading while you exercise. By the time you stop exercising and take a reading, your heart rate may already have dropped.

Also, exercise machine sensors give you your pulse rate, which is the opening and closing of an artery at a specific point. They do not measure heart rate, which is the electrical signal of the heart sent by the Sinal Atrial Node. See the question above regarding the palpitation method.

Finally, exercise machine sensors have no capability for programming exercise specific to you and your goals. They are a one-size-fits-all kind of technology.

Heart Rate Zones and Benefits

	TARGET ZONE	INTENSITY % OF HRmax	EXAMPLE DURATIONS	PHYSIOLOGICAL BENEFIT / TRAINING EFFECT
5	Maximum	90-100%	Less than 5 minutes	Benefits: Increases maximum sprint race speed Feels like: Very exhausting for breathing and muscles Recommended for: Very fit persons with athletic training background
4	Hard	80-90%	2 - 10 minutes	Benefits: Increases maximum performance capacity Feels like: Muscular fatigue and heavy breathing Recommended for: Fit users and for short excercises
3	Moderate	70-80%	10 - 40 minutes	Benefits: Improves aerobic fitness Feels like: Light muscular fatigue, easy breathing, moderate sweating Recommended for: Everybody
2	Light	60-70%	40 - 80 minutes	Benefits: Improves endurance, helps recovery Feels like: Comfortable, easy breathing, light sweating Recommended for: Everybody
1	Very light	50-60%	20 - 40 minutes	Benefits: Improves overall health and metabolism Feels like: Very easy for all bodily functions Recommended for: Novice exercisers, weight management, active recovery

Source: Polar Electro, Inc 2011

Excerpts from my First Book, 'Welleness'

Productivity Return on Investment (ROI)

"I don't have time."

"Yes, you do. You simply need to make it a priority."

I've heard people claim they don't have time to do things, literally, thousands of times (I've been there myself). It's the simplest and most widely used excuse out there. And that's what it is – a pure, 100% excuse. We make time for the things that are important to us, plain and simple.

What's important to you?

We all start with the same finite amount of time: 24 hours in a day; 168 hours in a week. And we choose how we invest this time.

From a productivity standpoint, ROI refers to how much you're accomplishing in a given period of time or with a certain amount of energy (both discussed later). The best way to think about ROI is to think about how we used to learn in school. We had a set period of time that was blocked off (semesters or quarters, and time during the day) to learn a given subject. When we had this singular focus, we had a great ROI. We got a lot done in a comparatively short period of time.

Why don't we approach our lives the same way?

I believe one of our fundamental problems is that we are spread too thin. We try to do too many things in too short a period of time. Consequently, we don't end up doing anything very well. Almost everything is given less than our best effort because we're too preoccupied and distracted to give it our singular focus.

Time ROI

Most people will discuss ROI (Return on Investment) in regards to financials; how much return ($$) we can expect on a given investment ($$). We can look at time the same way.

The difference is, of course, that we all start on a level playing field when it comes to the investment of time. There are no rich or poor; everyone begins with the same amount.

> "We all start with the same finite amount of time; but some choose to invest it more effectively than others."

Do you not have time to exercise? No time to eat well? No time for this person or that activity? No time to sleep?

Perhaps we need better financial planners, which is essentially the role of a coach or personal trainer. They tell us how to invest our time to get the biggest return. If we do not have anyone advising us, at the very least, we need to manage the investment well ourselves. If we find that we don't have time for many of the things that are important to us, something has to change.

Now, it's not my place to tell you how to prioritize your life. I believe in individual priorities and values and I believe in our right to be able to choose them. So, however you decide to structure your life and spend your time, just realize that you have time for everything you want to do.

I've been lucky to work with many different types of people and I've seen firsthand how prioritizing time and energy can provide dividends. Some of these people completed Ironman triathlons and others have lost weight and toned up, but both required a healthy time commitment and an assessment of priorities.

Energy ROI

In the previous paragraphs we discussed how to properly invest time – but what about the investment of energy? There are some tasks that drain lots of time but very little energy (watching TV, surfing the internet, cooking) and things that require lots of energy (driving in bad weather, presenting at work, chasing your kids). The key is to match our energy output to the task-specific demands.

Let me explain: energy is a less quantifiable term than time. We don't know how much energy we have, but we all know the subjective difference between when we have it and when we don't.

<blockquote>
"The key is to match our energy output to the task-specific demands."
</blockquote>

The two most universal ways of renewing your energy are exercise and sleep. But there is a third way to renew energy, and it is by participating in things you find intrinsically enjoyable. The easiest way to identify things you find intrinsically enjoyable is to answer the question, "What would you do if you had all the money and free time in the world?"

The answer to this question is what you find intrinsically enjoyable.

Most people think, I would go to a Caribbean island and lay on the beach, but would you really? Wouldn't that get old after a while? I think this is a default answer not because it's a means of energy renewal, but because it's a way to deflect from the responsibilities and obligations of our everyday demanding lives.

So, while sleeping and exercise are the two best methods of renewing energy, this becomes nearly irrelevant if you continue to waste it on things that, in the grand scheme of life, do not matter.

> "We need to stop wasting our energy
> on things that do not matter."

We should stop wasting our energy getting angry with the person in front of us who is driving slowly. We should stop getting frustrated at the long lines when we go to Target and Wal-Mart. We should stop worrying about the weather forecast for the weekend.

Each of these three examples is an energy drain. None of them are in our control. Directly, and possibly practically, there's nothing we can do about them. I suppose we could stop driving, shop at a more expensive store where there will be better service and less people, or stay inside where the weather doesn't matter. Each of these three could be perceived as "fixes," but they aren't really fixes at all – they're band-aids.

Let's look at another example—my distaste for doing dishes. Now, my family never had a dishwasher growing up so I was forced to manually wash and dry the dishes for the first 18 years of my life. It was traumatic! So, perhaps that's why even the small act of rinsing the dishes and putting them in the dishwasher nowadays annoys me. And I used to simply throw the dishes in the sink...just so I could worry about them later. After I'd do this for a while, the dishes would start to pile up and, eventually, I'd have to rinse them ALL at once and put them in the dishwasher.

Big deal, right? Well, the total amount of time it took me wasn't any greater doing it that way vs. rinsing them as I was dirtying them. But the ENERGY drain of watching the dishes stack up in the sink would always bother me. I hated looking over there, knowing eventually I'd have to take care of them.

Isn't this the way we approach a lot of things in our life? We put things off and put them off until, finally, it gets to a point where something HAS TO be done. And doing it this way requires a lot more energy in the long run.

The true fix is to manage things as they come at us, be slightly uncomfortable now so we can be comfortable later and control our reaction to the events and how much energy we expend.

These simple fixes would allow us to have much more energy for the things that really matter: friends, family, profession (assuming you enjoy your job), faith, and personal development. It all starts with managing our energy.

Take Home Points and Action Plan

Answer the question, "If I could do anything right now, what would it be?" Next, identify whether you're doing anything to move towards that answer.

If the answer is NO, brainstorm ways you could reprioritize your time and energy to move in that direction. Are you able to identify any areas in which you're wasting energy that, if freed up, would give you more energy to move towards what you really want to be?

If the answer is YES, is there anything else you can do with your time and energy to accelerate the process? Be creative!

Repair. Rebuild. Recover.

Our body is all about routine. We can train our body not only to fall asleep faster but we can also improve our efficiency of sleep.

Sleep can be looked at two ways:

- ✓ How long does it take you to fall asleep?
- ✓ How is the overall quality of your sleep after you've fallen asleep (do you wake up during the night, do you dream, etc.)?

Sleep Quantity

The most common cause of struggling to fall asleep is overthinking. Almost always, this stems from thinking about what happened today or thinking about what is going to happen tomorrow.

The two primary emotions that keep you awake at night are guilt and worry. Guilt stems from feelings about something that has already happened in the past and worry stems from things you believe may happen in the future. On some level, almost all of your overthinking can be tied back to these two emotions.

"Guilt and Worry are USELESS Emotions."

The most efficient way to cure the curse of overthinking is to determine ways to *rid yourself of it.* So, before going to bed, stop for a moment and think about if you have anything weighing on your mind that may keep you awake. If you do, what can be done to alleviate this before you go to sleep? Maybe it's a phone call or an email. Maybe it's one last overlook of a presentation. Maybe it is organizing some of your things so you don't feel rushed in the morning. Or maybe it's prayer.

Any of these things can help give you peace of mind. Do not discount the importance of a last-minute activity/ritual before going to bed. A calm mind leads to a calm body.

If there is *nothing* you can do about it, why are you worrying? Or why are you feeling guilty? It's done. Finished. Set in stone. There is no need to dwell on something that is unchangeable. Better to start fresh and move forward with calm, more positive thoughts.

Sleep Quality

- ✓ *Do you wake up in the middle of the night?*
- ✓ *Is your sleep restless?*
- ✓ *Do you wake up and not feel rested?*

What we do before we go to bed can help our sleep quality. When we sleep poorly, it most likely means we're not achieving "REM" sleep, which stands for Rapid Eye Movement. REM sleep is when you dream and is crucial to the secretion of certain hormones that help your body rebuild, recover, and restore itself.

There are some simple points that can improve your sleep quality.

- ✓ ***Avoid alcohol.*** I know that probably sounds harsh to some of us, it's a proven fact that alcohol leads to poor sleep *quality*. Yes, it may help you fall asleep faster, but if we wake up the next morning still feeling tired, does it really matter? At the very least, limit the amount of alcohol you have at night to one or two drinks.

- ✓ ***Limit caffeine****, especially at night*. No coffee, tea, soda, or energy drinks. Caffeine is a stimulant and will not only affect how long it takes you to fall asleep, but also how long it takes you to relax into deep sleep.

- ✓ ***Limit sugar****, especially at night*. Sugar can give you a short jolt of energy by spiking your insulin levels but, similar to caffeine, it will undoubtedly affect your sleep quality by making it more difficult for your body to achieve REM sleep.

- ✓ ***Be careful of over-hydrating before going to bed.*** Excess water will cause you to wake up in the middle of the night because you have to go to the bathroom, thus disturbing the sleep cycle.

- ✓ ***Don't exercise before going to bed.*** This is probably a no-brainer for 99% of the population but exercise, while great for the body and metabolism, causes a spike in appetite and energetic endorphins – not what you want when you're trying to fall asleep.

Take Home Points and Action Plan:

Guilt binds you to the past; Worry binds you to the future. As my mother always told me:

"Yesterday is history, Tomorrow is a mystery, and Today is a gift – that's why they call it The Present."

So do *whatever* you can to rid yourself of guilt and worry *before* you go to bed and then let it go. You'll sleep better for it.

Be Comfortable Being Uncomfortable

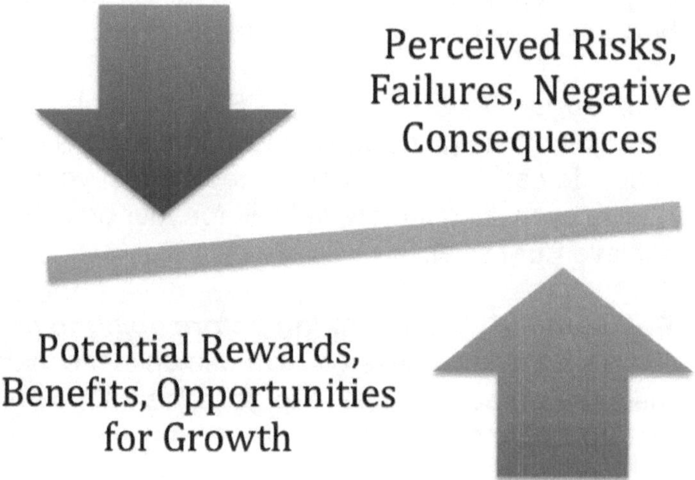

I've worked with and studied hundreds of high achievers and one thing mentioned repeatedly is how we have to be slightly uncomfortable with our life if we're going to achieve anything great. We have to step outside of our comfort zones. We have to stretch ourselves. It's a non-negotiable characteristic of super achievers.

Why is this?

When we're challenged we are forced to grow. We rise up and meet the challenge or we fall short and live to fight another day.

To grow, we must be pushed beyond our own physical or mental limitations. Great rewards only come from great risks.

In the fitness world, we follow a simple principle of Stress + Rest = Adaptation. In a way, any type of challenge can be looked at this way. By "stressing" (i.e., stepping outside our comfort zone) and then recovering, we grow stronger than we were before. We get closer to reaching our potential - to being the best we can be. But it's very easy for us to coast and to not create this stress. We'd rather stay where we are. With no stress comes no growth...and no positive adaptation.

> "When you are challenged you are forced to grow.
> You HAVE TO grow or you don't meet the challenge."

I've also noticed that super achievers describe learning much more from their "failures" than from their successes. Failures are nothing more than a stepping stone to success. And every time a super achiever fails, they know they're one step closer to doing it right the next time. They take accountability, don't take failure personally, brain storm solutions, and use it as an opportunity for growth.

Low achievers, on the other hand, usually attribute failure to an excuse, their own inadequacy, or an insurmountable obstacle outside of themselves. The fear failing (see previous chapter) and their ego is bruised when mistakes are made. Each time they fail, they're that much more hesitant to put themselves out there and try again (think of business sales, diets and relationships). Instead of moving closer, failure actually moves you further away from the end goals.

Surprisingly, many people don't know the story of Colonel Sanders (but I'm betting you've seen or eaten at a *Kentucky Fried Chicken!*). He started the business at age 65 so he already had Father Time working against him. But that's not even the most remarkable part. When he was traveling around, trying to sell his *finger lickin' good* chicken recipe, he receive 1009 no's before he received his first yes.

Let me repeat that – *one-thousand and nine* no's before he received his first yes! How many of you would have persevered and continued on after the first thousand? After the first hundred? After the first TEN? That's why there are very few Colonel Sanders. Low achievers will never fail enough to get there. Super achievers fail repeatedly and learn from the mistakes until they find success.

The Difficulty of Challenges

The tough part about challenges is that we often see a black-and-white dichotomy of success OR failure. Nothing in between. No shades of gray. Thus, we are reluctant to attempt challenges because of the *perceived* risk of potential failure.

Think of lifting weights. If you want to get stronger, a basic premise of strength training is to lift a weight until muscular failure, or to the point that you cannot lift the weight another time (even if you tried). Doing this challenges the muscle and forces it to grow and build stronger than it was before. Do this enough times and you'll have a positive adaptation.

Every area in our life can be looked at the same way. But challenges ourselves in other areas is difficult because of:

- ✓ Finding a challenge that is difficult enough to stretch you (or make you uncomfortable)
- ✓ Finding a challenge that isn't so difficult you view it as unrealistic and unattainable
- ✓ Finding a challenge that is meaningful to you and will keep you engaged

Each of these is important in its own way. A meaningful and engaging challenge is critical. Without it, there's no way you'll see it through to the end. Viewing a challenge as unrealistic and unattainable comes back to attitude. Nothing is unattainable unless you believe it is. Again, whether you think you can or think you can't, you're right.

Of the three, finding the appropriate challenge to stretch you, and make you slightly uncomfortable, is probably the most difficult. Most people who have never run before would probably not be advised to sign up for a marathon. It would be too much stretch, too much stress, and too uncomfortable. Of course, you may know people who have done this, but they would have combated the huge stretch with a glass-half-full attitude and an incredible meaningfulness.

> "Too often we see the dichotomy of success OR failure. Nothing in between. No shades of gray."

Again, this is where individuality comes into play and only you know what challenges you'll respond the best to. In general, a very small percentage will respond to extremely lofty challenges, whereas a much larger percentage will respond to challenges that are slightly beyond our comfort zone and don't seem too daunting.

Effort and Expectations

Somewhere along the line high expectations got a bad wrap and we started avoiding them. Why?

Because high expectations come with a greater sense of responsibility and obligation, and a greater chance for failure. Based on the before-mentioned societal conditioning that we're all susceptible to, most people are not built to embrace (or withstand) the added pressure of these expectations. But couldn't we also see high expectations as a compliment of our abilities and an opportunity for greater success?

I've worked with many high level athletes and you hear them asked all the time, "How do you handle the expectations (the media, the fans, your previous successes) that are placed on you?" They almost always come back to the same answers – "I focused on my preparation. I focused on the things I could control. I focused on the process. I *did not* focus on what other people were saying and what other people expected of me."

There are two problems with expectations. First, expectations are almost always based on outcomes (here we go again). This is because outcomes are our most tangible measure of "success." It's all that people can see. This is why it was discussed extensively in regards to attitude.

Second, we don't like expectations because somebody else places them on us. It feels more threatening when someone else imposes their expectations on us. The number one rule of goal setting is that you come up with your own goals, expectations and standards of performance.

The surefire way to beat this is to always have higher expectations of yourself than anyone else can possibly have of you. Adopt your own psychology of excellence. Embrace your individual high standards. Own it.

(You're probably wondering how this can be...especially if you're a high level athlete and people expect you to win every game or make every shot)

Again, the answer lies in *effort,* or once again controlling the set of the sails. Effort is 100% in your control. There isn't anything anyone can do about it. And, I promise, if we focus on working hard and giving 100% effort to the things that are important to us in life, we'll never give a second thought to expectations. They won't matter. We will have done our best and that's all anyone can ask. We can look in the mirror with no regrets.

> "Adopt your own personal psychology of excellence that is higher than anyone else can put on you."

Still, this is easier said than done. Effort is very difficult to measure and effort doesn't always translate to positive outcomes. Sometimes we try our absolute hardest and still fall on our faces. And because the outside pressures and expectations usually come from the results of outcomes, it is tough to escape them. But regardless of what area of your life comes with expectations, if you're able to step away and say that you gave your best effort, you will feel good – no matter the result.

Take Home Points and Action Plan

Two simple, open-ended questions:

✓ *What are your expectations of yourself for today? This week? This month? This year? Are these higher or lower than the expectations others have of you?*

How are you going to make it happen? What are you committed to? What is your personal psychology of excellence? Write it.

Surround Yourself with People who Pull You Up

There are two kinds of people in this world: those who pull you up and those who pull you down. Which type of person would you rather associate with? Would you rather spend time with people who are negative and do not challenge you, or those that can make you better?

Studies have proven that whom you surround yourself with is as big a determinant of your own success as anything else. In fact, almost all studies say that your health, wealth and happiness will be the average of the five people with whom you spend the most time. Choose your close friends and peer group wisely. They'll likely dictate your future.

I love this quote from Jim Rohn:

"You must constantly ask yourself these questions: Who am I around? What are they doing to me? What have they got me reading? What have they got me saying? Where do they have me going? What do they have me thinking? And most important, what do they have me becoming?

Then ask yourself the big question: Is that okay?"

Who Pulls You Up?

People who pull you up usually have one of the following characteristics:

- ✓ They have infectious positivity and energy
- ✓ They have something you want
- ✓ They challenge you
- ✓ They are someone you can learn from
- ✓ They are someone you respect and admire
- ✓ They share similar values to your own
- ✓ They have a great sense of humor

I would be willing to bet that almost every "special" person in your life fits into one of these categories. But how great would it be if there were even more of these people? When our "circle" consists of people who all pull us up, we cannot help but improve—in all facets of our life. What a great thing!

> "There are two kinds of people in this world: those who pull you up and those who pull you down."

Who Pulls You Down?

I typically refer to people who pull us down as "energy vampires." They literally suck the energy out of you. Instead of giving you energy, they take it away.

I do not like to focus on negativity but it is important that it be addressed here. Unfortunately, we all have people in our lives that pull us down. These people can be coworkers, family or friends. Sometimes we may fail to realize who they are. We just get "used to it."

The bottom line with these people is they don't bring anything to our table. They come to mooch off us. They take our energy away. They drain us of positivity and belief. We walk away afterwards feeling the same, or often times worse, than we did before. They CONDITION us.

The irony in all this, and it relates to the chapter on being comfortable, is that many of us would rather be comfortable and potentially feel worse, than be uncomfortable and feel better. The comfort level keeps us coming back for more. We don't want to shake the tree.

Now, I understand that these situations can be complicated. It's difficult to choose our coworkers or our bosses, and our friends and acquaintances. And it's impossible to choose our *families*. Each of these situations can be complicated and I'm not advocating we all quit our jobs, find new friends, and disown our relatives.

> "If someone pulls us down, is there something
> we can do to pull them up?"

What I am saying is it's important we recognize who these people are and to not let them affect us. Be aware of it and create a buffer against it. If someone is going to punch you in the stomach and you don't see it coming, it can easily knock the wind out of you. But if you see it coming, you are able to brace yourself and it doesn't hurt as much. It helps even more if you pay the price of admission for six-pack abs :)

Pulling Other People Up

In the essence of making everyone who reads this book, better, it's also important to take the time to put ourselves in someone else's shoes. If there is someone in our life that doesn't necessarily pull us up; is there something we can do to pull them up? Can *we* be the person that challenges them and spurs them on to be better? Can we inspire, as well as be inspired? Can we get these people to see the world through our glass-half-full perspective?

I'm a firm believer that we were put on this planet to pull other people up. We were all meant to inspire. We all have that ability. Sometimes, we don't feel like we do but I can tell you from personal experience that the fastest way to feel better about yourself is to help someone else feel better.

I'm not saying we can do this with everyone. The person would have to be willing to change for us to be able to pull them up. Sometimes people are more comfortable in their own sadness. But it's worth the effort. These reciprocated relationships make everyone better.

Take Home Points and Action Plan:

What are the most important areas of growth for you? Examples:

Spiritual	Is there someone in the church that you can grow closer to? Or a bible study?

Health	Who do you know that embraces a healthy way of life? Can they help you do the same?

Professional	How would you like to grow in your career? Who knows something about it and could help you?
Personal	Do you have a hobby you'd like to take up? Or something about the way you conduct yourself that you can improve?
Mental	Who has a mental attribute that you don't have (attitude, confidence, productivity, focus, etc.)? Is there something you can learn from this person that would enhance your mental ability?

Try to identify a person (or better yet, people) who can help you in your most important areas. Ask for help...most people are willing if you have the courage to ask.

About the Author

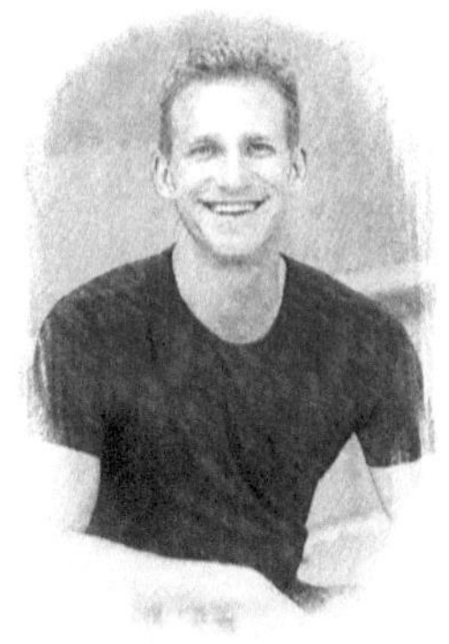

SCOTT WELLE is a #1 international best selling author, speaker and founder of Outperform The Norm, a global movement that coaches athletes and business leaders to raise their game and perform at the highest level.

While the rest of the competition is playing not to lose, Scott teaches people to play to win. His proprietary "Commit / Attack / Conquer" formula ensures people fall asleep at night knowing they are making the most of their precious days on this planet. For this, Fox 9 in Minneapolis-St Paul has called him a *"Motivational Expert."*

Scott has always loved sports but felt he underperformed early in his career by not mastering the "mental game." After graduating with his Master's degree in Sport Psychology, he made it his life's mission to coach people to higher levels of performance and not let others repeat his mistakes. Throughout this process, he's realized how the same mental principles that allow athletes to be successful will allow business leaders to achieve exceptional results, and this formed the foundation for Outperform The Norm.

Now, Scott's eight best selling books, articles, videos and podcasts inspire hundreds of thousands of people worldwide and students in over 35 countries have taken his online courses. He is an adjunct professor at St. Olaf University and serves on advisory committees of three national level organizations. He regularly coaches top performing executives, sales professionals and entrepreneurs, as well as elite athletes, all with one common goal: to OUTPERFORM.

Scott enjoys pushing his own physical and mental limits, completing five Ironman triathlons, 29 marathons, R2R2R (47 miles back and forth through the Grand Canyon) and a 100-mile ultra marathon run. He is very close with his brother, Jason. Together they "plod" at least one marathon together each year, laughing the whole way.

Please visit him at ScottWelle.com.

Also by Scott Welle

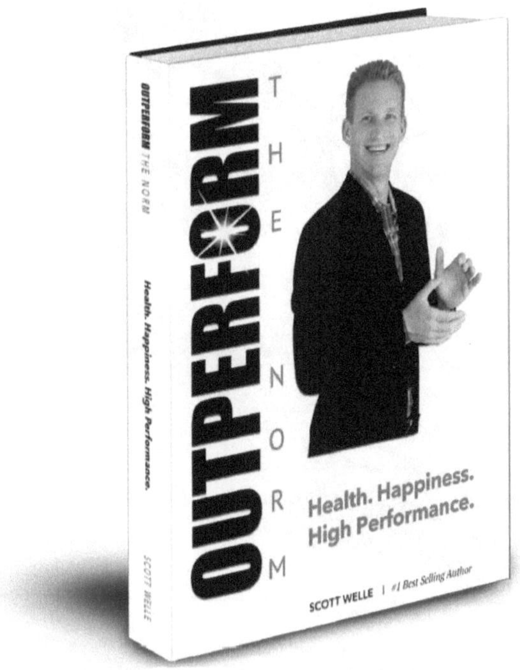

OUTPERFORM THE NORM

Health. Happiness. High Performance.

OutperformTheNorm.com/books

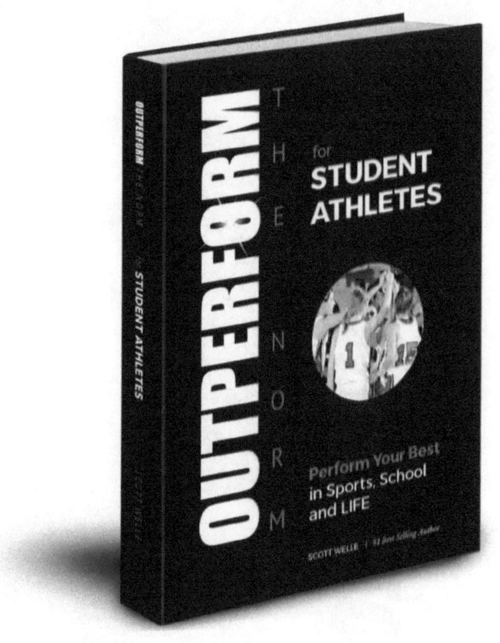# OUTPERFORM THE NORM
for Student Athletes

Perform Your Best in Sports, School and LIFE

OutperformTheNorm.com/books

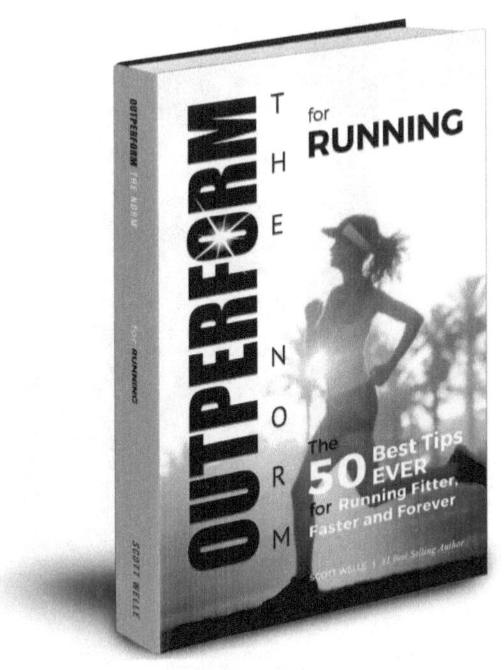

OUTPERFORM THE NORM
for Running

The 50 Best Tips EVER for Running
Fitter, Faster and Forever

OutperformTheNorm.com/books

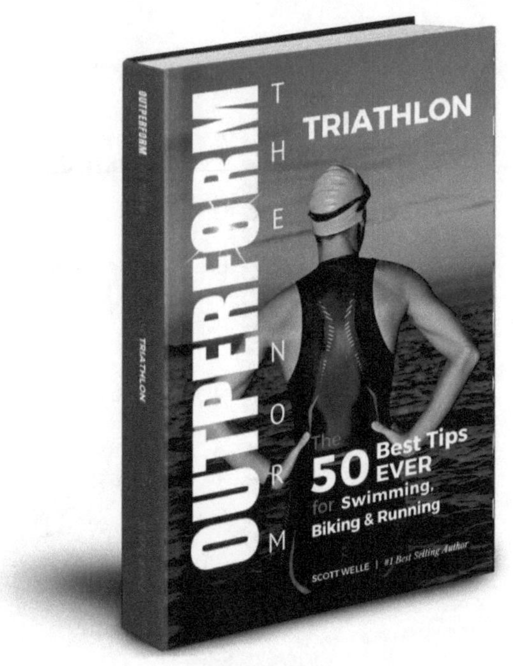

OUTPERFORM
THE NORM
TRIATHLON
The
50 Best Tips
EVER
for Swimming,
Biking & Running
SCOTT WELLE | #1 Best Selling Author

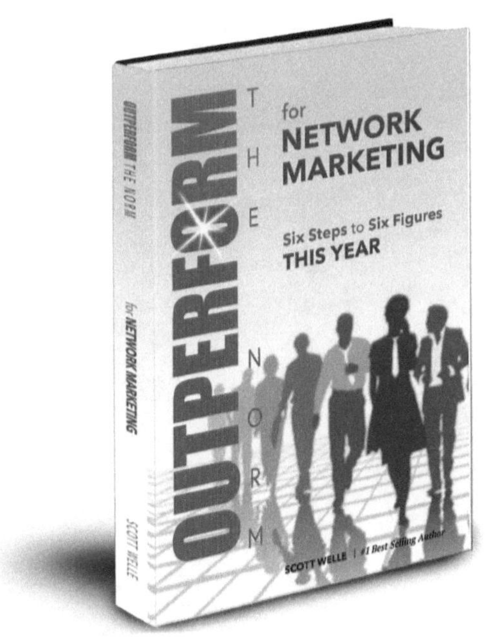

OUTPERFORM THE NORM
for Network Marketing

Six Steps to Six Figures This Year

OutperformTheNorm.com/books